The
Complete
Prenatal Water Workout
Book

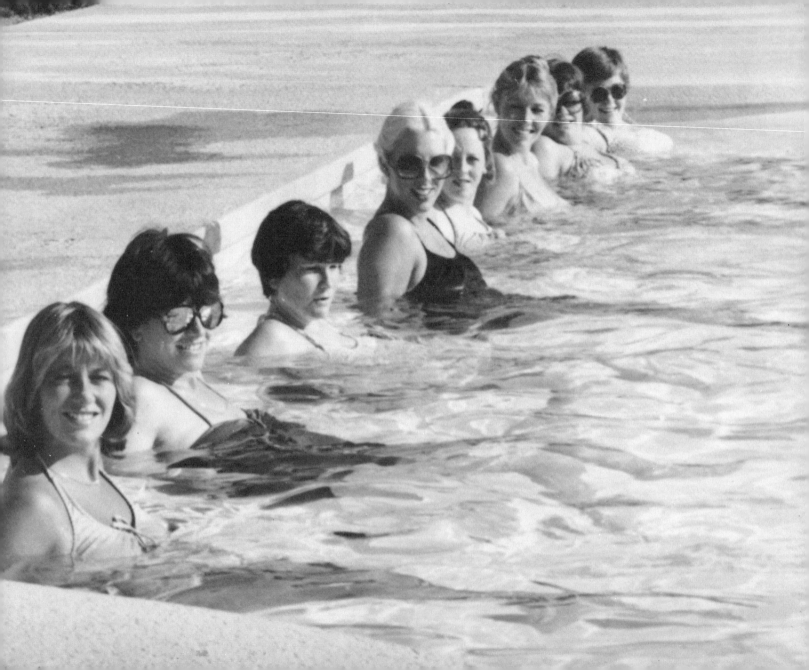

The Complete Prenatal Water Workout Book

Based upon the Successful *Watercise While You Wait* Program

Helga Hughes

Photographs by Ken Hughes

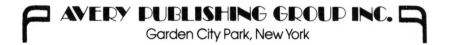

AVERY PUBLISHING GROUP INC.
Garden City Park, New York

The ideas, procedures, and suggestions contained in this book are based upon the experience of the author, and are not intended as a substitute for consulting with your physician. All matters regarding your health require medical supervision.

Cover Design: Martin Hochberg and Rudy Shur
Cover Photo: Terry Cuffel
Text Photos: Ken Hughes
In-House Editor: Joanne Abrams

Library of Congress Cataloging-in-Publication Data
Hughes, Helga.
    The complete prenatal water workout book.

    Bibliography: p.
    Includes index.
    1. Pregnancy. 2. Aquatic exercises. 3. Prenatal
care. I. Title.
RG558.7.H84 1989   618.2'4   88-7441
ISBN 0-89529-306-4 (pbk.)

Printed in the United States of America

10 9 8 7 6 5 4 3 2 1

Contents

Dedicated to my daughter Susan
and her son Steven,
my blessed grandson.

Acknowledgements

First and foremost, to those "moms-to-be" who attended my early classes. Their support and encouragement planted the seed that grew into this complete prenatal water workout.

To all the lovely models who gave willingly of their time to pose for the photographs used throughout this book.

To YWCA, YMCA, city parks, and swimming school directors who have made *Watercise* a part of their planned activities.

To all those in the childbirth-related field—especially obstetricians, midwives, and childbirth educators—who recommended *Watercise* to their patients.

To my dear friend, the late Jean Janas, who gave so much to motherhood, and whose influence over my personal life will never be forgotten.

To Neil J. Shernoff, M.D., for his endorsement of *Watercise*, and for his invaluable review of my first manuscript to this edition.

Last, but most important, to Marilyn Kieffer, C.N.M., for sparing some of her precious time to write the foreword to this book.

Preface

"Watercise While You Wait" is a stress-free prenatal water exercise program designed to physically and mentally prepare the mother-to-be for childbirth.

The idea for this program first occurred to me when my daughter Susan was pregnant with her first child, now my much-beloved grandson, Steven. Susan complained to me of never-ending exhaustion, swollen and aching feet, legs that felt as heavy as lead, and a persistent backache. Even though she spent a great deal of time resting, she experienced no relief. In fact, the prolonged periods spent lying down worsened matters by impeding circulation. Vital blood supplies to her legs and feet were being reduced, causing a feeling of heaviness in the legs, together with painful cramps. Obviously, decreasing Susan's activities was not the answer. It seemed to me that increasing her activities in a manner that would make her feel lighter and more mobile was the best solution. Furthermore, because her physical problems were tending to produce related emotional problems, I felt that such a regimen would not only help relax her body, but also her mind, as well as help her achieve that all-important early and positive bonding with her child.

Naturally, I was greatly concerned about my daughter's well-being, and I tussled with the problem of what she should do and how I could help her. Finally, I recalled the great success I had experienced over five years earlier when I was the Recreation Director at Ahwatukee, a retirement center near Phoenix, Arizona. It was there that I had been faced with a similar problem. At Ahwatukee, however, I had not dealt with a young woman whose pregnancy was causing physical and emotional distress, but with senior citizens who had worked hard for most of their lives and were finally looking forward to the comforts and pleasures of retirement. Unfortunately, the ravages of time, work, and worry had taken their toll in many cases, and the residents were often incapable of carrying out the exercises they so desperately needed if their retirement was to be healthful and fulfilling. In some cases, the strength of muscle groups in their arms and legs barely equalled the pull of gravity; in others, afflictions such as arthritis cancelled any muscular development that had been achieved. To put it in a nutshell, for one reason or another they were unable to *energetically* move their arms and legs against the pull of gravity.

Ultimately, I realized that I must *remove* the effects of gravity, but since I could not transport everyone into the weightlessness of outer space, I took them into the water. The natural buoyancy of water effectively reduced their apparent weight to just a few pounds; yet, at the same time, the water provided an acceptable resistance against which their arms and legs had to work. In fact, the water was better than outer space would have been, because for exercise to be effective there must be resistance, and the water was providing it in a gentle way. Slow movements produced a minimum of resistance; fast movements, more. Moreover, the resistance was experienced in *all* directions—not just up and down, as with gravity.

I formulated a set of enjoyable exercises that the residents of the center could handle, and found that even after a full hour they felt no discomfort. In fact, they felt remarkably fresh and rejuvenated after each class. As time went on, the physical condition of the participants improved, often with a lessening of pain from afflictions such as arthritis, allowing those whose activities had been restricted to return to a full life.

With the memories of those earlier days at Ahwatukee in my mind, I went to work on a new program—not only for my daughter's benefit, but also for the benefit of my grandchild-to-be. I borrowed exercises from my earlier program and modified them when necessary to suit the special needs of my daughter, and I developed new ones designed to strengthen those parts of her body specifically associated with childbirth. Then I decided to give some of the exercises names that were related to the arrival of the new baby, thereby strengthening my daughter's motivation by reminding her of her goal: the birth of a beautiful child.

When we began the program, Susan was skeptical. She had bought several prenatal exercise books, but had found that the exercises caused stress, imbalance, or awkwardness. I explained how the buoyancy and gentle resistance of water would remove the stress and allow her to balance easily while performing the exercises. We persevered until she became enthusiastic and then—miraculously—began to feel better. The aches and pains were gone, and her positive attitude towards childbirth was reinforced.

The Complete Prenatal Water Workout Book

I soon realized that I was at the threshold of a truly comprehensive prenatal exercise program that could benefit *every* pregnant woman. When I thought about the many expectant mothers who might be helped by these exercises, I knew that they would not all be alike. There would be very young mothers-to-be, and there would be those in their middle age. Some would be single, but the majority would be married. Some would be carrying their first child, while others would be adding to an existing family. Many of them would be healthy, and some very fit, but a minority would be sick. Then there would be those accustomed to regular exercise, and others who would not be in good physical condition. Finally, there would be those anticipating a Cesarean birth.

Clearly, no one program could cater to everyone, but I decided that the exercises would be designed to give the maximum benefit to the majority, *without the stress or risks that accompany a high-pressure workout.* My aims were specific: to enhance posture; to strengthen the muscles used in labor and birth; to strengthen the muscles used for child care; to vitalize the body so that there would be a rapid return to prepregnant condition; and to limit weight gain to a healthy level (between twenty and thirty-five pounds).

While I was confident that the first four of my aims could be achieved by an exercise program, I doubted that a few hours a week of such exercise would control weight gain. Recollections of my own unhappy experience with the "pickles-and-ice-cream" urges that afflict pregnant women suggested that weight would have to be controlled as much by diet as by exercise. This called for an approach that would repress pregnancy-related eating urges. I decided that a blending of the motivational aspects of a positive mental attitude with the stretching and toning exercises I had formulated would achieve the desired results, as well as encourage the adoption of a happy, gentle, and loving disposition during those special nine months in a woman's life when her emotional well-being is most vulnerable.

As with all things, time and effort produced a route over the mountain of problems that stood between my early plans and the creation of a workable program, and on April 5, 1982, I taught my first organized program at Arizona's Mesa Family YMCA. Over one hundred mothers-to-be attended these classes, and just about each one of those lovely ladies wrote to me after giving birth to say how the program had helped her. The Mesa YMCA had become the birthplace of *Watercise.*

Since that time, more and more exercise and health professionals have turned to water for a solution to some of the problems of disease and infirmity brought about by the aging process. Many YMCA and YWCA branches throughout the nation now offer water exercise programs for arthritic sufferers, as well as for people with back problems, and I have found that the exercises are not dissimilar to the ones I first formulated at Ahwatukee. Furthermore, hospitals throughout the world have long utilized the buoyancy of water in the treatment of those stricken with various degrees of paralysis.

Today, a great number of physical education curricula include water exercises—albeit, the name has been stylized to "aquacalisthenics" or "hydrocalisthenics"—and many leaders in physical education have praised the all-round benefits of water exercises. Their remarks are typified by those of Ray Bussard, head swim coach at the University of Tennessee, who had this to say about exercising in water: "This type of muscular development loosens the body, giving the person a greater ease of movement, creating muscles along the exterior frame that pull in the bulges." Don Gamgriel, an Olympic coach, got right to the nub of the matter with his comment: "The water's buoyancy removes the stress and strain associated with land exercises."

Although the first edition of this book offered the same underlying philosophy and the same basic exercises as this new edition, its primary purpose was to supplement class instruction. The second edition differed little from the original.

The evergrowing demand by pregnant women who wish to work out on their own, either with their families or in privately organized groups, was the main reason for creating this third edition of *The Complete Water Workout Book*. The many new photographs and an increase in descriptive detail make it easier to follow the exercises, and the expansion of the text preceding the exercise sequence provides for a better understanding of the unique concept of *Watercise*. This edition also includes new exercises that can be performed in the shower and tub, as well as new, fun water exercises that the expectant woman and her partner can do together.

This book remains one that is essentially about an exercise program for pregnant women. But because of the importance of a positive mental attitude and because pregnancy is so special in so many ways, it became necessary to add discussions of family- and work-related stresses, diet, life in the womb, and intrauterine bonding. However, in recent years, knowledgeable authors have written many books on the subject of childbirth, often exploring or comparing hospital procedures and prepared childbirth techniques. Furthermore, diverse methods of childbirth preparation are taught by numerous national and international organizations, embracing alternative birth centers, home birth, breastfeeding, midwives, labor support people, hospitals, and obstetricians. In short, this book was not designed to *replace* the many excellent forms of childbirth education that are available today. Rather, it was created to meet the needs of the mother-to-be who wants an exercise program that is both effective and stress-free.

My feelings as a mother—and as a grandmother—go out to you, a future mother, cherishing the hope that you will benefit from this book as much as my own daughter did. During the months to come, be encouraged by the experiences of the many who have *Watercised* through their pregnancy with positive results. Believe in yourself.

Foreword

Pregnancy provides a marvelous time for a woman to focus on the wonders of her body as it nurtures the miracle within her womb by making daily changes in order to keep in harmony with the ever-growing new life.

The life-giving properties of water reinforce a fundamentally beneficial exercise program by supporting the body and easing movement, while the sensation of weightlessness allows a pregnant woman to feel graceful.

When I first talked with Helga, I was impressed by her holistic concept of exercise incorporating breathing procedures, relaxation, and positive mental attitude. I believe it is vital to view pregnancy as a process that involves the total person, and that all aspects of healthful living be adopted during pregnancy. The reinforcement of this holistic point of view through an exercise program is refreshing and rewarding for me, a health care provider who believes that the individual has unlimited potential in the achievement of optimum health, especially during pregnancy.

Since that first meeting with Helga, I have been fortunate in realizing a dream that had been with me for many years—the establishment of the Birth & Family Center of Phoenix, the first free-standing birth center in this city to be planned, directed, and staffed by certified nurse-midwives. Many of the women who have come to my birthing center have *Watercised* during their pregnancy, and I have found them to be better prepared—mentally and physically—for the birth of their child than those less fortunate women who did not *Watercise.*

Just as necessity is the mother of invention, need and love are the two basic motivating forces in the creation of ideas, concepts, and new life. How appropriate that an exercise program for pregnancy—the ultimate expression of love—was born of a daughter's need and a mother's response with love.

Thank you, Helga, for that loving response to the needs of your daughter. As a result of it, you have given hundreds of pregnant women the opportunity to enhance their health, as well as the health of their unborn children. With this third edition, there will be an unlimited number of others who will also benefit.

Marilyn J. Kieffer, C.N.M., P.C.
Birth & Family Center of Phoenix

Motherhood

Whether she is wearing a gown of lace,
    With pearls from the depths of the sea,
Or a well worn old frock made from muslin,
    With wild flowers adorning her hair.

Whether she walks down the aisle of a church
    Resounding with organ and song,
Or stands under a cathedral of trees
    With bird song on flower scented air.

Every bride makes her commitment
    With stars in her eyes,
Believing marriage to be true love.

Whether her first born arrives in this world,
    Midst satin sheets and skilled physicians,
Or in the simple room of a cabin
    With but her husband by her side.

Whether the babe is born to inherit
    Untold wealth and a famous name,
Or be that babe just one more of many
    To inherit the earth far and wide.

Every mother makes her commitment
    With tears in her eyes,
Knowing motherhood to be real love.

Chapter One
You, Your Body, and Your Baby

This book is essentially an exercise program for pregnant women. The exercises themselves are unique in their utilization of the buoyancy of water and in their targeting of those areas of the body that are most affected by pregnancy and birth. The postpartum period, too, will be made more comfortable by the *Watercise* program.

You will have a greater appreciation of the *Watercise* workout if, before beginning to exercise, you learn about the physical changes that take place during pregnancy. While such preparation is important for everyone, it is most important for the woman who is expecting her first child, and who therefore may not have a clear-cut understanding of the physiology of pregnancy and birth.

This chapter, which focuses on the important topics of good posture and sound prenatal nutrition, begins the discussion of pregnancy.

YOUR PRIORITIES

You are in charge of your pregnancy. Once you accept this fact, you should begin to adjust your lifestyle to suit both your own needs and those of your baby. Take into consideration your job, your physical activities, your leisure activities, any mentally fatiguing tasks you must perform, and any unnecessary demands that may have been placed on you by others. You do have choices, and you do have the right to do those things that best suit your new condition. It is a condition that the majority of women experience only a few times in their lives, and one that requires but nine miraculous months to fashion a whole *new* person from a microscopic seed.

THE PHYSICAL YOU

Your body will surely change as your pregnancy advances, ranging from the obvious swelling of the belly to subtle changes, such as the exertion of pressure on those organs surrounding the uterus; the placement of added weight on legs and feet; and a shift in the body's center of gravity. However, except for the tummy, you will not have to lose your figure. Indeed, with proper exercise and a positive attitude, you can look even better, because the added maturity and love, and the fulfillment of a happy pregnancy will grace your face and make your eyes shine.

The *Watercise* exercises have been designed to help those areas of your body where changes will take place, as well as those parts that will be indirectly affected by the changes.

Posture

In *Have Your Baby, Keep Your Figure*, Dr. M. Edward Davis, former Medical Director of the American Association of Maternal and Child Health, and Edward Mausel, former Director of the American Physical Fitness Research Institute, state: "Posture should be your first consideration." Unfortunately, posture is a much used but little understood word. Essentially, posture is ideal when the spinal column is not curved out of shape and the body is in a state of equilibrium. What few people realize is that *bad* posture must involve bending the spine in *two* places, not just one. In the case of a well-proportioned person who is neither overweight nor underweight, slumped or rounded shoulders that cause curvature of the upper spine will always be counterbalanced by the stomach being pushed forward as the spine takes an "S" shape in order to maintain balance. In the case of an ill-proportioned person, such as someone with a stomach enlarged by overeating, the "S" shape of the spine usually starts at the bottom, with compensation taking place at the top.

Without compensatory redistribution of weight in order to regain equilibrium, the only way a person can control improperly balanced weight is by locking the feet and leg muscles. Obviously, if a person with good posture were to have a heavily laden tray thrust into her hands while she was in an upright position, she would have to either put a foot forward to create balance, or lock her feet and leg muscles.

Therefore, when a woman who has good posture becomes pregnant, she has two choices: she can counterbalance the increasing weight in her womb by slouching, thereby creating the spinal "S," or she can keep her balance by using muscle power to retain good posture while sitting, standing, and walking. Since distortion of the spine often leads to health problems, a pregnant woman *must* learn to use muscle power— which she will probably have to develop. The Stork Walk on page 30, the knee bends on page 32, and all the leg exercises in this book will fill this need. The woman whose posture was *bad* before pregnancy will need to work harder to correct it by exercising more frequently and by doing more repetitions of each exercise. In either case, the need for countering imbalance will not cease after delivery. During and after the postpartum period, imbalance will be present when the baby is in the mother's arms or on her hip as she goes about her daily activities.

When to Start Exercising

During the first trimester of pregnancy, the fetus grows to a length of less than six inches. This causes no obvious weight gain or obvious enlargement of the associated organs. Thus, posture is not affected. However, the time to begin exercising for the maintenance of good posture is *before* your swelling abdomen puts unaccustomed weight on your stomach muscles, and *before* your balance is upset. Similarly, early exercising of the chest muscles will help prevent the breasts from sagging as pregnancy advances and the breasts become larger from the growth of milk-secreting glands. (See exercises on pages 38 and 40.) Also, early exercising of those pelvic muscles associated with the uterus and the birth canal may help reduce labor and delivery time. (See the Water Kegel on page 58.)

Studies point to the great advantages of starting a stress-free exercise program *early* in pregnancy, and most health professionals recognize the need for limited exercise *throughout* pregnancy. Many women *Watercise* right up to their last week, and their reports on the benefits of the program indicate that *Watercise* not only eases labor and delivery, but also speeds a return to prepregnant condition, with little loss of skin tone and muscular elasticity.

Although the benefits are clearly greatest for those women who are able to begin exercising in the first trimester, benefits have been experienced by those only able to begin in their second, or even third, trimester. In any exercise program, the frequency of performing the exercises, as well as the speed of carrying out repetitions, has a direct impact on the degree of benefit obtained. Thus, as long as the late starter avoids strain and fatigue, she may wish to exercise more frequently, with faster repetitions.

Diet

During pregnancy, diet plays a more important role in your life than ever before, affecting both your physical and emotional well-being. No longer are you eating just for yourself. No longer can you get by with makeshift meals hastily prepared from convenience foods. The microscopic miracle of life that started within you on your first day of pregnancy grows by the hour, and if that growth is to be sustained until you deliver a fully developed, healthy baby, you must control your diet.

In his introduction to *Eating for Two*, Dr. Tom Brewer, director of a prenatal nutrition education program at the Contra Costa County Medical Service between 1963 and 1976, states: "Mother and baby are one biological unit. Whatever affects one, affects the other. Nourishing the mother is the only way to nourish the baby."

What you put *into your body* is what you put *into your unborn baby's body*. Thus, the calories you consume to create those extra pounds of "baby weight" should have real nutritional value, and should not be empty calories like those found in junk food.

An inadequate intake of nutrients will require protein to be burned for energy, resulting in protein deficiency in both mother and baby. As the essential building blocks of cells, protein should be an integral part of your expanded diet. Preferably, the protein should be derived from fish, poultry, eggs, dairy products, and legumes, with some limitation placed on red meats.

Your expanded diet should also include the other nutrients needed every day of gestation to keep you and your baby in good health. They are the vitamins A, B complex, C, D, and E; the minerals calcium, sodium, and iron; fats; and carbohydrates. All of these nutrients are vital for a successful pregnancy, and all are needed in quantities greater than normal.

Aim for whole, natural foods. Whenever possible, eat raw vegetables and fruits, as they will help prevent the constipation that so often afflicts pregnant women. Eliminate refined sugars, candies, sugar-laden sodas, fried and fatty foods, and all foods containing additives.

Nutrition is by no means the central theme of this book, and my advice to the pregnant woman is to follow the diet recommended by her medical advisor, or—in the absence of such advice—to follow the diets given in specialized pregnancy nutrition cookbooks, such as *Eating for Two* by Isaac Cronin and Gail Sforza Brewer. Both you and your child will reap the benefits of your efforts.

Non-Food Items and Drugs

It was once thought that the placenta was a magic barrier that prevented any harmful substance in the mother's blood from being passed on to her baby. Unfortunately, this belief was false. Obstetrical pharmacologists now agree that virtually all substances injested by the mother are transmitted to the baby. This includes drugs, nicotine, caffeine, and alcohol. These substances—except for those medications taken with the consent of your obstetrician—should be avoided during pregnancy.

It is now a widely accepted fact that the toxic substances in cigarette smoke are harmful to humans. These substances do pass through the placenta and can restrict fetal growth, increase the risk of premature birth and stillbirth, and cause a higher incidence of sudden infant death syndrome. In addition to these health hazards, the offspring of heavy smokers may also experience behavioral problems.

Alcohol in any quantity also has a toxic effect on the fetus, with effects ranging from lower-than-normal birth weight to mental retardation.

Caffeine is present in coffee, tea, chocolate, and a number of soft drinks. Various studies have shown a connection between caffeine consumption and problems such as premature birth, low birth weight, and stillbirth. As a safe level of caffeine consumption has not yet been determined, it is advisable to eliminate or reduce caffeine intake during pregnancy.

Finally, drug addicted pregnant women give birth to drug addicted babies who, from their first day of life, experience the torment of withdrawal.

Tobacco, alcohol, coffee, and other non-food items have no nutritional value, and pose many risks. By eliminating them from your life—or, at the very least, reducing your exposure to them—you not only will help ensure normal fetal development, but will greatly improve your own physical and emotional well-being.

YOUR COMMITMENT

Childbirth may well be the greatest challenge you ever face, and it is up to you to assume responsibility for what is to be the most creative event in your life.

Once you have selected your medical advisors, trust them. Have them explain to you and your husband anything you do not understand, and have them guide you in selecting the best available childbirth education and preparation classes. Then attend these classes regularly, if possible with your husband.

Incorporate into your life the vital elements of exercise, good nutrition, knowledge, and confidence; and learn the techniques of relaxation, proper breathing, and energy conservation. You will glean many of these skills from your *Watercise* program, and they will help prepare you to assume an active and fulfilling role in the birth of your child.

The Complete Prenatal Water Workout Book

Chapter Two
The Importance of a Positive Mental Attitude

In the previous chapter, considerable importance was attached to the maintenance of physical health. Of no less importance is the need to adopt a good mental attitude. In all walks of life, a positive attitude is essential for success, and the need is perhaps greater if a successful pregnancy is to be achieved. This chapter deals with this need.

PREPARING THE MIND

The *Watercise* exercises have been designed to physically prepare you for labor and delivery. However, much of your effort may be wasted if you are not mentally prepared. While there is no simple program that can guarantee your emotional well-being, a positive mental attitude will help you to have a happy and healthy nine months of pregnancy.

In order to reinforce your awareness that there is a real, new life within you, it may be worthwhile to consider the Chinese belief that life begins at conception. Thus, a child is already nine months old at birth. In more recent times, this ancient belief was affirmed in the book *Life Before Birth* by Ashley Montagu, noted anthropologist. Montagu states: "The basic fact is simple: life begins, not at birth, but at conception."

Preparation for the birth of your child should begin as soon as your pregnancy is confirmed. Developing the right mental attitude from the outset is as important as making an early start with the right exercises and the right diet.

The efficiency of the reproductive system in a *normal* woman's body is such that under *normal* conditions, nothing will hinder the orderly progression of pregnancy, labor, and birth. From the start, when the fertilized cell first starts to split and multiply, its needs can be met with pure food and oxygen supplied by way of your blood stream, and with the protective aura of love that flows from you. Thus, if through strength of mind you can achieve and maintain physical fitness and avoid indulging in non-food products, you will protect your baby and be rewarded with a healthy and contented child.

It is essential to create an image of joyful motherhood within your mind. This mental picture, which anticipates your coming experience, should be an image of all that is beautiful. The body is the vehicle of birth; the mind the driver. It was your mind that developed the passion and desire first needed to fulfill your biological role in the conception of a new life. It is your mind, too, that must help your body to mold and fashion the child you are carrying.

INTRAUTERINE BONDING

Over two thousand years ago, philosophers and physicians such as Aristotle and Hippocrates believed that the female is *more* than just a factory in which the physical child is made and delivered. In recent times, scientific studies have supported this belief. *Your mind* is one of the chief influences on *your baby's developing mind.* Through your thoughts, you will help to create your child's first indelible memories—memories that may affect his ideas and actions in later life. It is, therefore, as important for your baby as it is for you to have only beautiful and positive thoughts about yourself and your *unborn* child, thereby imprinting on the precious mind of that child only expressions of love: a love not blighted by undertones of fear. Your fear of childbirth can be as harmful to your baby as it can be to you. In your case, the chief effect will be to disturb the neuromuscular harmony of labor, causing muscles to tighten into uncomfortable spasms when, in fact, they should be relaxing. In your baby, the effects may be of longer duration. This link between the mind of the pregnant woman and the mind of the developing fetus is known as intrauterine bonding.

Acceptance of the phenomenon of intrauterine bonding has come full circle. A thousand years ago, the Chinese had prenatal clinics that were as much involved with emotional care as with physical care. Five hundred years ago, our ancestors believed that a mother's emotions could be transmitted to her unborn child, and care was taken to shield pregnant women from unpleasant experiences. Earlier in this century, however, the idea that prenatal experiences can influence the child's personality would not have been tolerated.

Obviously, facts about prenatal life are difficult to acquire. Those facts that are available have been deduced from the way a baby's heart beats and his body movements change when the mother is subjected to stimuli such as noise, or to emotional shock.

Many experiments and studies were conducted in postwar Europe, when malnutrition, fear, and fatigue were commonplace. One of the studies, confirming that intrauterine bonding does take place, was conducted by Dr. Monika Lukesch, a psychologist at the Constantine University in Frankfurt, West Germany. She followed the pregnancies of two thousand women, and in a dissertation published in 1975, concluded that the mother's attitude during pregnancy had the greatest single effect on the child's early personality.

This study, and many others that are referred to by Montagu in *Life Before Birth* and by Dr. Thomas Verny in *The Secret Life of the Unborn Child*, have helped support the idea that a woman who *wants* her pregnancy, who feels a strong love for and attachment to the forming child, and who experiences a comfortable, unworried pregnancy and delivery, is likely to have a well-adjusted child.

Verny classifies the links between mother and unborn child as either *sympathetic (extrasensory) communication* or *physiological communication*. Factually, little is understood of the former; thus, the results of studies currently being performed by the American Association for the Advancement of Science are eagerly awaited. As far as physiological communication is concerned, it is known that hormonal releases triggered by such emotions as anxiety and fear can pass through the placenta to the fetus. Both Montagu and Verny stress, however, that only a *continual* assault of anxiety-produced hormones can be dangerous. Minor, transitory worries will not endanger the child's welfare.

Enough evidence has been accumulated to indicate that the emotional scarring of children can often be traced to persistent negative emotions or stressful events flowing from mother to child in one form or another during gestation. Therefore, a mother-to-be should avoid exposure to unnecessary stress, and should make those who share her daily life aware of the effects of unpleasant experiences on the newborn.

YOUR MOST IMPORTANT ROLE

While you will play many important roles throughout your life, the one you assume during pregnancy is one of the most important, because you are actually living out two lives. For the sake of that second life, you must expose yourself to the best possible outside influences. Read good books on pregnancy and childbirth (refer to the Recommended Reading list on page 83); attend childbirth preparation classes; and, whenever possible, share these experiences with your husband.

Ideas, whether generated by your mind or imposed on you by the outside world, do control your life, be they positive or negative. It is up to you to be the skilled operator who can control them to your advantage. Pattern yourself after the woman who displays happiness as a complete person as well as a mother-to-be. Let your "cup runneth over" with joy, happiness, and fulfillment. And should you meet another mother-to-be who is unblessed, burdened with problems, and age-worn before her time, share with her the beauty of your positive thinking program.

SUMMARY

The following summary of this chapter provides a quick reference for those readers who may wish to reinforce their positive thinking from time to time.

- Negative thoughts have a destructive effect on your life, whereas positive thoughts have a creative effect on your life. If you *think* you are well, you are likely to *feel* well. If you think of your pregnancy and forthcoming delivery as beautiful miracles, they will be experienced as such. If you *communicate* lovingly with your unborn child by thought, word, and action, the benefits to your child—and thus to you—will be limitless. If you train yourself to think only positive thoughts, your life and your child's life will be full and rewarding.

- Reach out for the support of your husband. Together, choose the type of obstetrical care that you feel is best suited for you, and then accept your roles as parents-to-be.

- Prepare yourself for childbirth, both through reading and through in-depth communication with your medical advisors. Obtain from them knowledge of all routine and non-routine procedures. Exercise the choices available to you, basing your decisions on the advice you have received and on the knowledge you have gained from books and childbirth education classes.

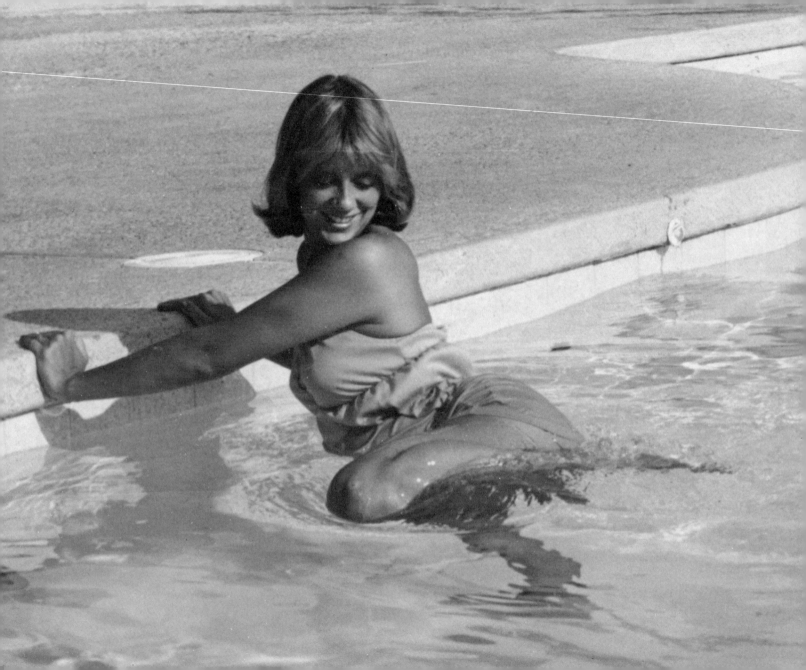

Chapter Three
Understanding the *Watercise* Program

That the approach to an activity is usually of great importance for success is well illustrated by the time spent by a professional golfer in addressing the ball. Although competitive golf is far removed from prenatal exercising, both strive for a goal, the achievement of which can be enhanced by taking the right approach. This part of the book deals with the steps that should be taken just before the action begins.

SELF-IMAGE

The unique aspect of *Watercise* is the blending of stretching and toning exercises carried out against the gentle resistance of buoyant water with the creative force of a positive mental attitude. Not only have I devoted a chapter of the book to this latter aspect, but the whole program was designed to encourage a joyful approach to motherhood. I place great emphasis on the need to foster an enhanced self-image and to create an atmosphere in which you can socially interact with other pregnant women in lightness of body and spirit.

Whether you *Watercise* by yourself or with others, that first positive step you took when you chose this exercise program will lead you all the way through a positive pregnancy.

The exercises presented in Chapters Five, Six, and Seven have been related to motherhood by name or by action whenever possible. Not only does this aid the process of intrauterine bonding, but it also gives greater meaning to each exercise. Many of my students have commented on how, for example, the names Stork Walk, Pray Keep My Bustline, or Rocking the Baby, helped them to visualize what an exercise *looks* like and what it does for the body, as well as intensifying their feelings of closeness to their unborn child.

REGULATING THE EXERCISES

Watercise movements should be gentle and stress-free and, unlike many modern workouts, they should *not* be done to the beat of music. Rhythm sets speed, usually constant and compelling, and you can be sure that the composer did not select the rhythm to suit the needs of your pregnant body. A musical beat that is too fast might easily *compel* you to try to keep up with it, thus forcing you into that gray area of exercising that requires careful monitoring of cardiovascular function.

There is no doubt in my mind that while music is a desirable accompaniment to some exercise sequences, such as high-speed aerobics, it can lure the mind away from that so important awareness of being *involved* with exercises, and can force the body beyond the limits of safety.

In order to both correctly set the speed at which you perform the exercises and determine the number of repetitions, an understanding of your own body is essential. If you have not exerted your body since your last calisthenics class in high school, then for your baby's sake *feel* your way into the program, resting whenever the need is apparent and stopping when you are truly tired. On the other hand, heavy exercisers may *think* the program is too easy, but they should first evaluate some principles. Frequently, exercise programs aim at either muscle development or an improvement of cardiovascular function, both of which are achieved by steadily increasing speed and difficulty. *Watercise* aims for neither, the object being to *tone* and *stretch* those muscles used during pregnancy, labor, childbirth, and child care.

POOL SAFETY

At this stage, just before we finally reach the water, some comment is necessary on pool safety and pool usage.

If you plan to exercise alone in your own pool, you should always have a family member or a friend watching your progress. Although this program is both safe and stress-free, some situation may occur that could cause you to lose your balance and fall, while an extremely hot day may cause you to feel faint. Anyway, it is not much fun to do things alone, so have someone with you—preferably your husband, who can work with you on some of the exercises. If you already have children, let them join you if they are good swimmers; otherwise, be sure they do not have access to the pool area. It is impossible to exercise *and* supervise young children at the same time. Naturally, if you have a friend who also is expecting, invite her to share the benefits of *Watercise* with you.

I must also caution you about the apparent change in body weight you will experience when you move out of the water at the end of an exercise session. When you finally climb the steps to leave the pool, you will feel gravity grab for you, dramatically changing a feeling of grace and lightness to one of overburdened weight. Whether you exercise in a group or alone, you should be aware of this phenomenon and anticipate its occurrence.

POOL USAGE

Watercise may be carried out in any pool. However, if you form a group and use a public pool, it would be wise to clear the program with the controlling authority.

In some public pools, the noise level created by excited children may distract you from successfully carrying out Retreat Time, a regimen that precedes the actual exercise sequence (see page 24). If this is the case, and you are aware of it beforehand, I recommend that you practice Retreat Time at home before leaving for the pool.

Pools vary considerably in design, causing some difficulty in following the exercise instructions to the letter. However, a measure of ingenuity will usually solve the problem. For instance, some pools do not have steps suitable for most of the leg exercises. The solution is to either use a paddle board to support your body or to hook your arms over the rail or wall in order to let your legs float up for the exercise.

BATHING SUITS

Some women who feel they must wear a tight-fitting garment for exercise—such as a leotard for aerobics—may dislike the feeling of exposure caused by wearing the garment. Undoubtedly, one advantage of exercising in water is that you can *look* graceful as well as *feel* graceful.

Maternity shops usually carry a wide range of fashionable bathing suits appropriate to all stages of pregnancy. Such a bathing suit will enhance your appearance out of the water and enable you to exercise in style and comfort in the water.

Chapter Four
Muscles

If you understand the workings of an automobile, you probably will be a better driver. Similarly, an understanding of muscles will probably improve your ability to exercise. Not only will such an understanding help prevent you from straining muscles through excessive or incorrect exercise, but it will give you an awareness of the muscle being exercised, enabling you to "tune in" to it. This chapter explains muscle function and describes the ways in which a pregnant woman benefits from prenatal exercise. It will allow you to fine tune your efforts.

MUSCLE GROUPS

Although the skeletal body is virtually covered with interlacing and interlocking muscles, for the sake of simplicity these muscles can be isolated into major groups. Sometimes a single muscle in a group is used or exercised, but more often than not, several muscles from one or more groups are used in conjunction with one another. Generally speaking, each muscle group relates to a specific part of the body, and it is wise for an exerciser to have some idea of exactly what is being strengthened, and what specific benefits will be achieved.

MUSCLE FUNCTION

In general, a muscle originates on a bone and inserts on another bone, often passing across a joint on the way. When tightened, the muscle contracts towards its origin, thereby pulling on the second bone and causing it to move. An easily understood example is the quadriceps group (the heavy muscles on the top of the thigh). This set of muscles originates at the front and side of the hipbone and at the top of the thighbone, extends down the thigh, passes around and into the kneecap, and finally inserts into the shinbone, just below the knee. When the quadriceps contract, the muscle action straightens the leg.

Some muscle groups, particularly the abdominals, work both to give support and to permit movement. The abdominals are composed of two groups—one on the left side and one on the right side—that work together to support the abdominal organs and aid in flexion of the trunk. This action is different from that of the left and right sides of the leg and arm muscle groups, which work independently to give movement.

LOWER LEG (CALF) MUSCLES

These muscles control all foot and ankle movements, and help rotate the lower leg. Exercising these muscles improves circulation, helping to eliminate leg cramps and varicose veins, and assists in the maintenance of good posture.

UPPER LEG (THIGH) MUSCLES

These muscles move the knee joint when squatting, sitting, walking, or running. Some of these muscles help hold the leg in or out, and help to rotate the leg. The muscles used to hold the legs apart are the posterior iliac muscles. When contracted (tightened), these muscles swing the legs out, pivoting at the hip joint. Exercising these muscles will help you to hold your legs apart for long periods during delivery without tiring. The adductor muscles, which pull the thighs together, are also important. If weak, they allow the pelvis to tilt downwards, causing the uterus to fall forward.

HIP MUSCLES

These muscles not only control many upper leg movements, including hip rotation, but also help stabilize the lower back. For this reason, these muscles are vital to good posture.

BACK MUSCLES

These muscles control a wide range of body motions, ranging from simple support to twisting and bending. They are important postural muscles.

ABDOMINAL MUSCLES

Think of these muscles as a four-way stretch corset, and although they always *feel* tight during pregnancy, do not be hoodwinked into thinking that they are in good shape. Like an overstretched corset, they will probably be out of shape after you have your baby—*unless* you exercise them. The abdominals hold the uterus in an upright position, are used during the pushing stage of delivery, brace the body when it is under stress, and help stabilize the lower back. Good abdominals are vital to good posture.

Although *Watercise* includes only one exercise specifically geared to strengthen the abdominals, almost every exercise in the book causes these muscles to flex.

SHOULDER AND CHEST MUSCLES

These muscles control the movement of the upper arms and the shoulder blades, and provide support for the breasts. Again, these are important postural muscles.

NECK MUSCLES

This complex group of muscles allows the head to move in almost any direction. Most important is their function in holding the neck straight for good posture. Weak neck muscles are one cause of the "S" shape of the upper spine often seen in people who have poor posture.

UPPER ARM MUSCLES

These muscles control the movements of the forearms, and are used in lifting and carrying.

LOWER ARM MUSCLES

These muscles are used for rotating the forearm as well as for most wrist and hand movements. All are vital to dexterity, and thus play an important role in child care.

PELVIC FLOOR MUSCLES

The three sets of pelvic floor muscles are the anal muscles (at the end of the bowel), the vaginal muscles (at the end of the birth canal), and the urethral muscles (at the end of the urinary bladder). Each of these muscles is a sphincter muscle (a ring), although they link together in a double figure eight, thus becoming virtually one muscle.

The pelvic muscles are the only support for the uterus, bladder, and rectum. Thus, good muscle tone is essential to prevent the lowering of these internal organs. After delivery, pelvic muscle exercises will restore proper tone.

This essential information about muscles will not only help you improve the quality of your exercising, but will improve your understanding of those parts of your body affected by pregnancy. Moreover, I hope it will let you "see" inside yourself, thereby enhancing your awareness of how your exercising will help your baby.

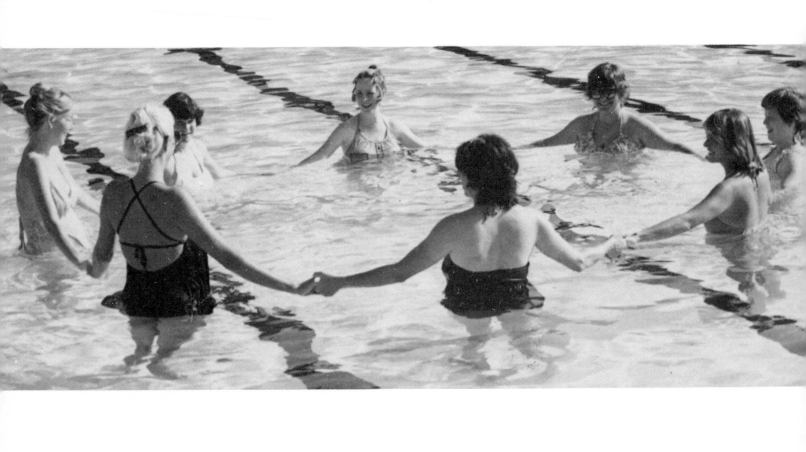

Chapter Five
The Exercises

At those locations where I have established a *Watercise* program, classes meet for two one-hour sessions a week. However, you will enjoy greater benefits by exercising three, four, or more times a week, so whether you are *Watercising* with others or on your own, try to *Watercise* as often as time and energy permit.

This chapter presents the basic *Watercise* routine—the essential part of the program. In addition to following this routine, you may wish to try the shower and tub exercises that are detailed in Chapters Six and Seven.

ILLUSTRATIONS

Each *Watercise* exercise is illustrated by a series of photographs. For clarity, these photos show the exercises being done *out of the water*. Also included with each exercise is a photo of an expectant mother at the time she attended a *Watercise* class, and in some cases the mother-to-be is partially out of the water for the same reason.

However, always keep in mind that a principle of *Watercise* is to keep the body submerged as much as possible in order to create buoyancy and help negate gravity.

EXERCISE VARIATIONS

The instructions for exercises 12, 13, 14, and 15 direct you to sit on the steps of the pool. In the event that suitable steps are not available, and you use the alternative method described on page 16, the exercise sequences should be changed to avoid fatiguing your back and arms. When using the alternative method, follow each "step" exercise with a "standing" exercise such as Family Circle (see page 44).

THE PROGRESS TABLE

The Progress Table on page 26 lists the exercises in the desired practice sequence, and shows the *suggested* number of repetitions that should be done at each *Watercise* session during the first four weeks of exercise. After this initial period, you may wish to further increase the number of repetitions—or you may wish to maintain the fourth-week level. Remember that the number of repetitions listed is only suggested, not mandatory. If you feel tired before the set number for an exercise is reached, you should stop and rest. Similarly, if you join a group of women who have already progressed beyond the first week, you should start out with the first week's recommendations (or less), and build up at your own pace. *Do not* feel obliged to keep up with the others—no one will criticize you for stopping. You are preparing for motherhood, not the Olympics.

RETREAT TIME

The benefits of both the physical and the mental aspects of *Watercise* will be enhanced if you begin each session with a relaxed body and a relaxed mind.

A tense body often stems from a tense mind, and a tense mind can stem from an unresolved problem. Having a tense mind is akin to having a dark cloud over your head, and it is this cloud that Retreat Time will help dispel.

Sit on a step of the pool with elbows behind for support and legs stretched out in front. Close your eyes and tilt your head back; then allow your legs to float to the surface of the water. Do not resist the buoyancy of the water. Let the water relax you, and say to yourself, "Let there be peace and harmony and trust and cooperation in my world, and let it begin with me." Then inhale slowly to the count of four before exhaling slowly, again to the count of four. Help the water to relax you even further by breathing slowly, deeply, and evenly. Let your body move with the water while you try to relax each muscle in your body. Start at your toes, focusing your mind on them to help them relax. Moving upward, relax each muscle group: the calves, the knees, the thighs, the abdomen, the chest, the shoulders, and the arms. Finally, relax your facial muscles, and under closed lids let your eyes move upwards. Allow your jaw to go slack and your tongue to sag.

When you are completely relaxed, the dark cloud of worry will float away. As you breathe slowly and evenly, in and out, and as your body rocks gently with the lapping of the water, the tension will leave your mind and you will be able to direct your mental energy to the child growing in your body. As your love enfolds the child, so the child's love will envelop you. Be aware of your miracle. Be aware that you, the child, and the child's father are as one, and look forward to the day when you will say, "Welcome to my world, little one."

Continue to breathe evenly and slowly. Keep your mind relaxed, knowing that the light of motherhood surrounds you and that the power of positive mental attitude protects you. With this knowledge, you will be able to change your thoughts from *limited* to *limitless*.

Once mind and body are relaxed, you can begin performing your exercises.

THE ERECT POSTURE

The erect posture is often referred to in the exercises. This posture can be established by standing with your back to a wall so that you are touching the wall with your heels, calves, buttocks, middle back, shoulders, and the back of your head. Your shoulders should be pulled back, and your chin should be tucked in.

PROGRESS TABLE

EXERCISES	REPETITIONS			
	Week			
	1	2	3	4
1 Full Deep Breathing	3	3	3	3
2 The Stork Walk (number of steps)	40	50	60	70
3 Loosening Up:				
Jogging (minutes)	1	1	2	2
Knee Bends (each position)	10	12	15	20
4 Preparing the Arms:				
Circles (number each way)	10	12	15	20
Breast Stroke	10	12	15	20
5 Happy Hands	6	8	10	12
6 Pray Keep My Bustline	6	8	10	12
7 Mother Jean's Bust Firmer	6	8	10	12
8 The Birds and the Bees	6	8	10	12
9 Family Circle	10	12	15	20
10 Baby's Wake-Up Stretch	10	12	15	20

The Complete Prenatal Water Workout Book

PROGRESS TABLE, *cont'd*

EXERCISES	REPETITIONS			
	Week			
	1	2	3	4
11 Rocking the Baby	10	12	15	20
12 Strampeln (minutes each way)	1	1	2	2
13 Bicycling (number each way)	20	25	30	40
14 The Tummy Tightener	10	12	15	20
15 The Leg Scissors	10	12	15	20
16 The Water Kegel	3	4	5	6
17 Side Bend Side (number each way)	10	12	15	20
18 Pelvic Water Rock	3	4	5	6
19 Leg Exercises (number each way)	10	12	15	20
20 The Cellulite Slayer	10	12	15	20
21 Pushing the Stroller (number of steps)	40	50	60	70
22 Full Deep Breathing	3	3	3	3
23 Happy Thoughts	See Exercise			

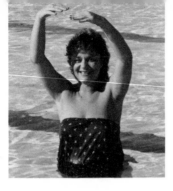

1 Full Deep Breathing

Purpose   Muscular activity absorbs oxygen. Deep breathing will provide you with the additional oxygen needed while exercising.

Preparation   Stand erect in waist-high water, with your legs eighteen inches apart and your hands held against the lower ribs.

Practice   Inhale slowly while raising your arms above your head in an easy sweeping motion, allowing your lungs to fill right up to the top of your chest. Exhale while leaning slightly forward and lowering your arms to a relaxed position. Repeat, this time holding your breath for a count of four when your arms are above your head. Exhale in the manner already described. This complete sequence should be repeated three times.

Pointers   Breathe in through your nose, and out through your mouth.

The Complete Prenatal Water Workout Book

"From the One came Two and from the Two all things are born."

—Tao Te Ching

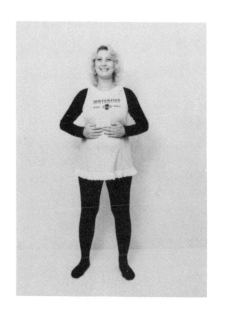

Hold hands against lower ribs.

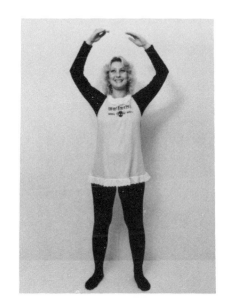

Raise arms above head.

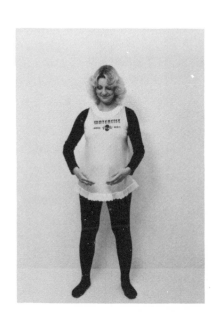

Lower arms to relaxed position.

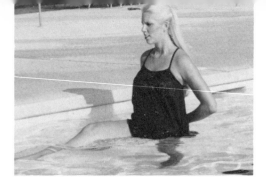

2   The Stork Walk

Purpose   The Stork Walk improves posture. The importance of good posture cannot be overemphasized. It prevents back pain and reduces fatigue. As an added bonus, good posture will enhance your appearance.

Preparation   Stand erect in water that is just above the waist. Clasp your hands behind your back, resting them above the buttocks.

Practice   Raise your right knee as high as is comfortable or until the thigh is parallel with the floor. Keeping posture erect by *not* leaning forward from the waist, straighten your leg and bring your foot down as you push forward with your left leg to complete the first step. Repeat with your left leg, and continue walking across the pool in a flowing motion for the number of steps recommended in the Progress Table.

Pointers   Walk tall to ensure that your shoulders do not slump forward.

"God could not be everywhere, so therefore He made Mothers."

—Talmud

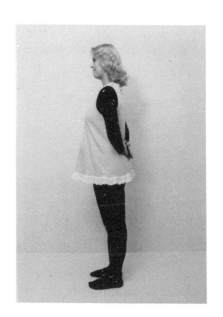

Clasp hands behind back.

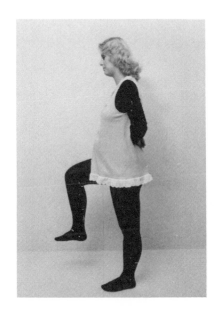

Raise right knee as high as comfort permits.

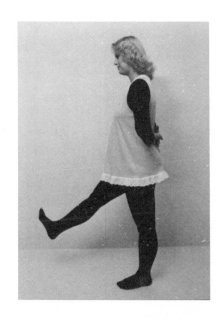

Straighten leg and push forward.

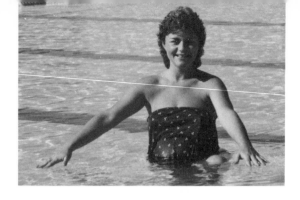

3　Loosening Up

Purpose　Warming up on land, or loosening up in water, is designed to lightly flex the muscles you will use for the principal exercises, thereby increasing the circulation of oxygenated blood to give muscles the energy they need. Loosening up will also help you avoid muscle cramps and tendon strains.

Preparation　Stand in waist-high water, with your feet slightly apart and your body erect.

Practice　First, jog in place, raising your knees as high as is comfortable. As you jog, hold your arms slightly forward from your body and rotate them by revolving them along their length. Do repetitions for the prescribed number of minutes. Next, stand erect with your feet turned out, heels slightly apart and hands on hips with thumbs forward. Rise onto your toes. Then lower and raise your body by doing half knee bends. Do the prescribed number of repetitions. Next, shift position so that your heels are well apart (about twelve inches) and your toes point inwards. Repeat the exercise in this position.

Pointers　When doing knee bends, place your hands on your hips with thumbs *forward* to help pull your shoulders back. This will enhance your posture.

"Into the woman's keeping is committed the destiny of generations to come after us."

—Theodore Roosevelt

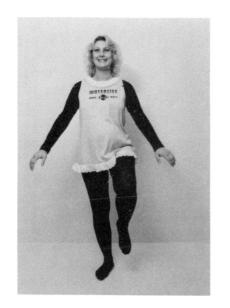

Jog in place.

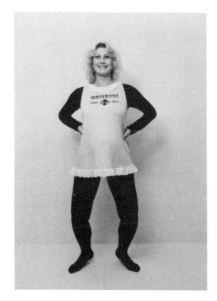

Do half knee bends with toes out.

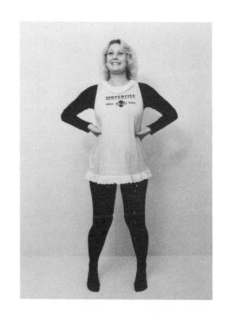

Repeat with toes turned in.

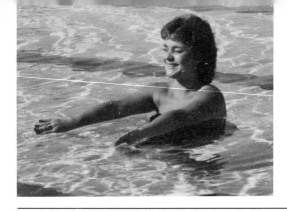

4   Preparing the Arms

Purpose By strengthening your arms, this exercise will prepare you to carry and care for your child after birth. As a bonus, this exercise strengthens chest muscles to help firm your breasts.

Preparation Stand erect in chest-high water, with your feet comfortably apart. Bend your knees to lower your body until the water is at shoulder level, and hold your arms outstretched sideways.

Practice Keeping your arms under water, swing them in a small circle for the prescribed number of repetitions. Then reverse direction and repeat the exercise. Maintain the bended-knee position and, with your back straight, practice the breast stroke arm movement by bringing the backs of your hands together in front of your chest, pushing them forward, and bringing them around in a sweeping movement—still under water—until they touch behind your back. Do the number of repetitions prescribed in the Progress Table.

Pointers Water must be at shoulder level so that arms are made to work against the resistance of the water.

> *"I think, at a child's birth, if a mother could ask a fairy godmother to endow it with the most useful gift, that gift would be curiosity."*
>
> —Eleanor Roosevelt

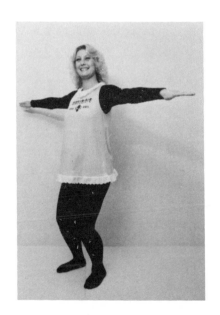

Lower body until water is at shoulder level.

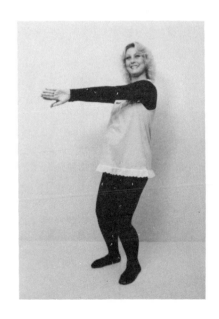

With arms extended, bring backs of hands together.

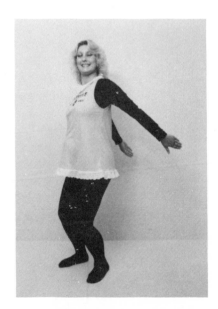

Practice breast stroke by sweeping arms behind back.

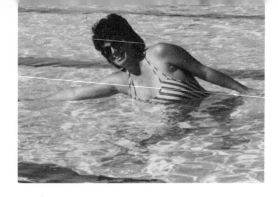

5   Happy Hands

Purpose   This exercise will make your fingers more nimble, enabling you to better care for your child's delicate organs, such as the ears. In addition, this exercise will help firm your waist.

Preparation   Stand erect in chest-high water, with your feet turned out and placed about eighteen inches apart. Let your hands hang loosely at your sides.

Practice   With fingers together, stretch your right arm forward. Count the thumb and fingers aloud, stretching each one wide apart on the count; then lunge towards the right, stretching your arms and fingers even farther. Return to the upright position and repeat the exercise with your left arm. Continue in accordance with the Progress Table.

Pointers   Lowering or raising your head will help you keep your balance while lunging.

The Complete Prenatal Water Workout Book

"Is there ever any particular spot where one can put one's finger and say, it all began that day, at such a time and such a place, with such an incident?"

—Agatha Christie

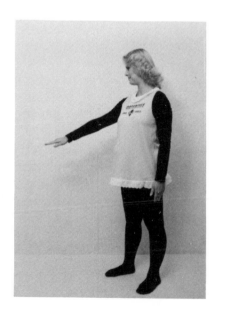

Stretch right arm forward.

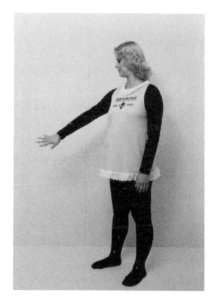

Stretch fingers apart, one by one.

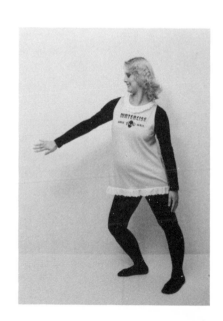

Lunge to right.

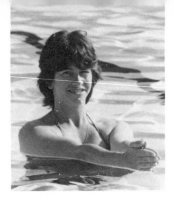

6   Pray Keep My Bustline

Purpose   This exercise strengthens the pectoral muscles, helping to maintain a good bustline during and after pregnancy. As a bonus, this exercise strengthens the thigh muscles in preparation for pushing during delivery.

Preparation   Stand erect in chest-high water with your back straight and your feet slightly apart.

Practice   Bend your knees to lower your body until water is at shoulder level. Bring your hands together in front of your body, with palms touching and fingers pointing *upwards* in a "prayer" position. Keep your forearms level with your shoulders. Exert pressure, and hold for a count of four; then relax. Stretch your arms forward, still at shoulder level, with palms together and fingers pointing *forwards*. Press together for a count of four, and relax. Next, straighten your legs and sweep your arms as far backwards as is comfortable. Hold for a count of four. Repeat this complete sequence in accordance with the Progress Table.

Pointers   When pressing your hands together in the first part of the exercise, imagine that you are compressing a small rubber ball between your hands.

"Infinite Love enfolds and protects me and my Child. Infinite Love sustains and strengthens us. My heart is full of faith."

—Unity Church

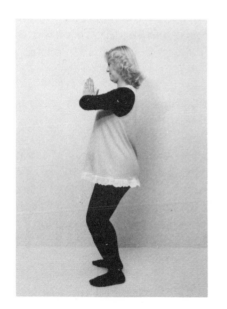 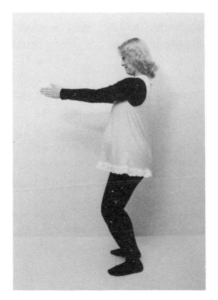 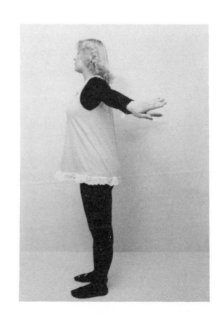

Bend knees and press hands together in "prayer" position.

Press hands together at full stretch.

Straighten legs and sweep arms backwards.

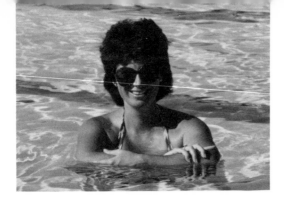

7   Mother Jean's Bust Firmer

Purpose   Another exercise aimed at the bustline, this one also increases the blood flow to the tissues under the breasts, which, it is believed, improves milk supply. This exercise will also improve your ability to hold your breath, which may be useful when pushing during delivery.

Preparation   Stand in chest-high water. With your back erect, bend your knees until the water is at shoulder level.

Practice   Lift your arms forward until your upper arms are parallel with the water, and grasp opposite wrists with hands, elbows pointing sideways. By pushing towards your elbows, and breathing in deeply, you will cause the muscles of your arms and chest to tighten. Hold for a count of four; then relax and exhale. Do this exercise in accordance with the Progress Table, feeling your breasts lift with each repetition.

Pointers   For maximum benefit, keep your upper arms level with the water.

"For to be a woman is to have interests and duties, raying out in all directions from the central mother-core, like spokes from the hub of a wheel."

—Anne Morrow Lindbergh

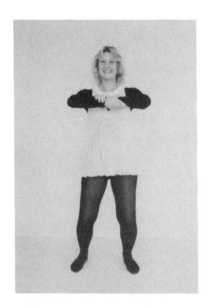

Grasp opposite wrists with hands,
and push hands towards elbows.

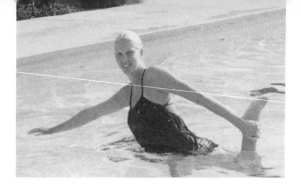

8 The Birds and the Bees

Purpose   This is designed to improve balance and to strengthen your leg muscles in readiness for all the standing a new mother must do. The exercise also flexes fingers to improve dexterity, which is so necessary when handling a small child.

Preparation   Stand erect in water that is above the waist. Place your feet a few inches apart.

Practice   Transfer your weight onto your right leg, stretching your right arm out in front to maintain balance. Lift your left leg backwards and up, grasping the ankle with your left hand to gently pull the foot in towards your buttocks, stretching the leg muscles. While maintaining your balance, stretch your right arm farther forward, rippling your fingers through the water. Repeat, using your other leg. Repeat this complete sequence in accordance with the Progress Table.

Pointers   Adjust your balance as necessary by bending or straightening the stationary leg.

"It was easier to give birth than to compete in the Olympics."

—Olga Korbut

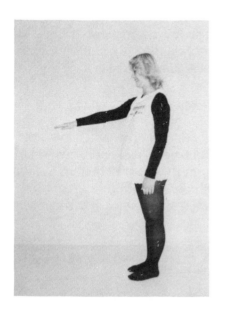

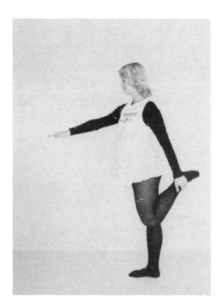

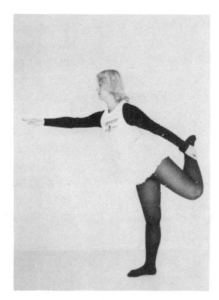

Put weight on right leg, and stretch right arm forwards.

Pull left leg up.

Stretch right arm farther forward.

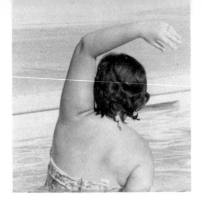

9   Family Circle

Purpose   Although you may already have a large *extended* family, the birth of your baby will create your own *personal* family circle. In this exercise, your arms form a circle to help you envision your baby. Family Circle will also strengthen your arm muscles, as well as those muscles that will help restore your waistline after birth.

Preparation   Stand erect in waist-high water, with your feet about eighteen inches apart.

Practice   Raise your right arm sideways over your head so that the arm and hand curve over your head, with your body leaning toward the left. Bring your left hand across your back, curving the arm upwards, so that your arms form the top and bottom halves of a circle. Now repeat in the opposite direction, with your left arm over your head, and your right arm behind your back. Repeat this complete sequence in accordance with the Progress Table.

Pointers   To exert the greatest pull on the muscles at the waist, avoid leaning forward as you bend sideways.

"I am a woman, mother and wife. If that means I am a sex symbol I am for it 100%."

—Sophia Loren

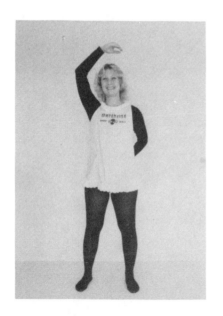

Position arms to form two half circles.

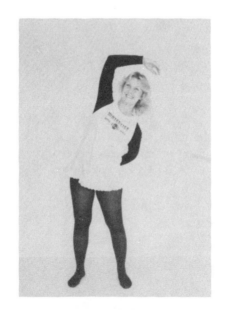

Bend to left.

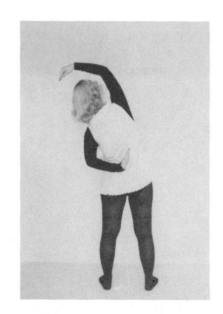

Maintain arm position throughout exercise.

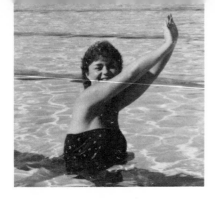

10   Baby's Wake-Up Stretch

Purpose   This overall stretching and toning exercise has the added benefit of firming the waistline.

Preparation   Stand erect in waist-high water, with your legs eighteen inches apart and your hands held close together in front of your chest.

Practice   While leaning to the right by bending from the waist, extend your arms sideways and up, straightening them as much as is comfortable, hands still held together. Return to the erect posture before reversing direction. Repeat this complete sequence in accordance with the Progress Table.

Pointers   To achieve the greatest pull on the muscles at the waist, avoid leaning forward when bending sideways.

The Complete Prenatal Water Workout Book

"Children are like hidden jewels a mother has the power to polish and present them to the world, or simply leave them dormant."

—Russian Proverb

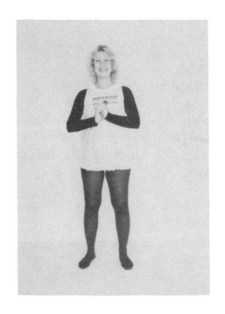

Clasp hands in front of body.

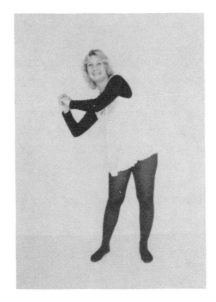

Lean to right, and stretch arms sideways and upwards.

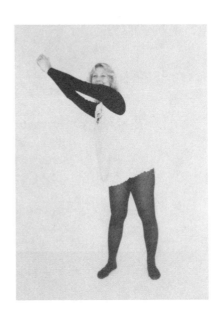

Continue stretch, straightening arms as much as comfort permits.

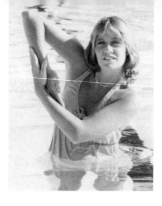

11   Rocking the Baby

Purpose   This combined waist-stretching and shoulder-strengthening exercise will also help you bond with your unborn child.

Preparation   Stand in waist-high water, with your legs eighteen inches apart and your body bent slightly forward. Hold your arms in a cradling position, with hands overlapping.

Practice   Swing your arms from side to side through the water, high enough so that each elbow lifts over your head. Turn your head in unison with arm movements, at the same time bending your knee so that the body lunges in the direction of the raised elbow. Smile as if your baby were already in your arms.

Pointers   When lunging, keep your heels on the floor to improve balance.

"My baby will have the career of a baby."

—Shirley Temple Black

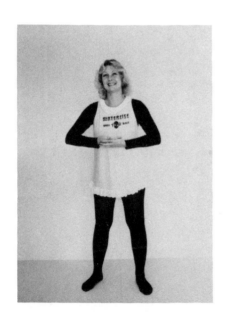

Hold arms in cradle position.

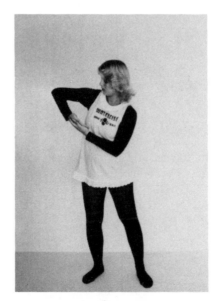

Swing arms from side to side.

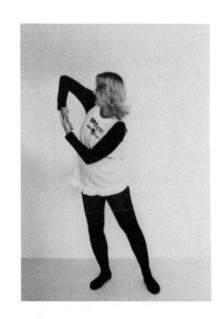

At top of swing, elbow should lift over head.

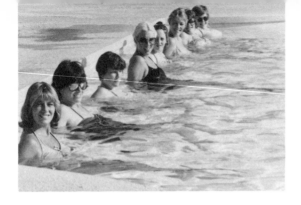

12 Strampeln

This German word specifically describes a baby's kick.

Purpose This leg-firming exercise also improves circulation.

Preparation Sit on a step. For added support, place your hands on the step, next to your buttocks. Allow your legs to float towards the surface of the water.

Practice Begin kicking as if doing the backstroke. Continue for the time prescribed in the Progress Table. Turn over, again with legs floating upwards, and kick as if free-style swimming. Continue for the time prescribed in the Progress Table.

Pointers Do not point your toes. Toe pointing often produces leg cramps.

"Each child carries his own blessing into the world."

—Yiddish Proverb

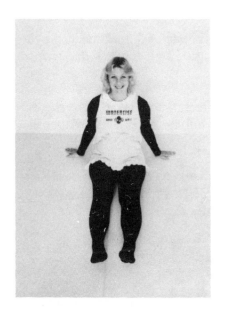

In sitting position, float legs to surface of water.

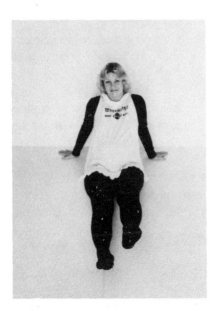

Kick as if doing backstroke.

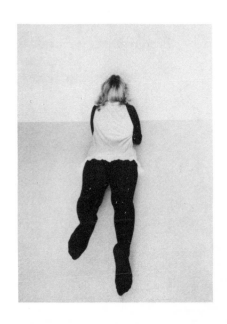

Roll over, and kick as if free-style swimming.

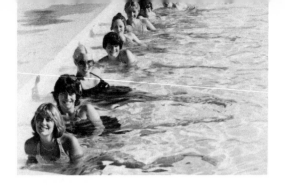

13   Bicycling

Purpose   This exercise strengthens the leg muscles and improves circulation.

Preparation   From the supported sitting position (*see* Strampeln on page 50), roll halfway over onto your right buttock, and allow your legs to float sideways towards the surface of the water.

Practice   Move your legs in a pedaling motion. Continue as recommended in the Progress Table, counting the repetitions when your left leg is at full stretch. Roll to the opposite side and repeat.

Pointers   To prevent cramps, avoid pointing your toes. The advantage of being on your side is that you can achieve larger pedaling circles with your feet. Be sure to keep your feet in the water at all times so that they will encounter continuous resistance.

"Taking joy in Motherhood is a woman's best cosmetic."

—Maria Montessori

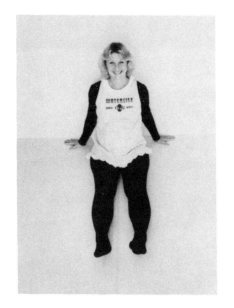

In sitting position, float legs to surface of water.

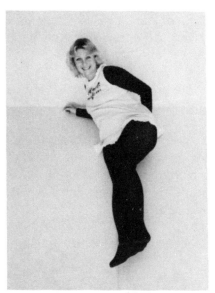

Roll over sideways.

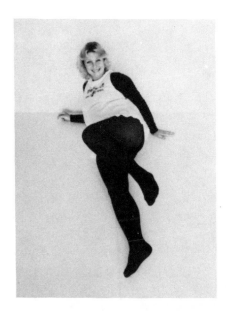

Move legs in pedaling motion.

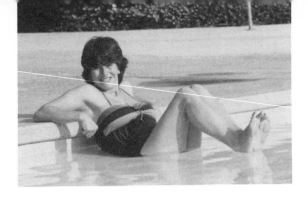

14   The Tummy Tightener

Purpose
As the name indicates, this exercise firms the abdominal muscles. These muscles must be firm to hold your uterus in the required upright position, to ease and speed labor and delivery, to improve posture before and after birth, and to hasten the recovery of your figure after birth.

Preparation
Sit on a step of the pool so that water is at bust level. With your spine straight, lean back a little, supporting your upper body by bracing your arms on the steps.

Practice
With your feet together and your knees bent, raise your knees towards your chest, as high as is comfortable. Straighten your legs while stretching them forward, level with the floor, before lowering them to the sitting position. Repeat in accordance with the Progress Table, inhaling on the upward movement and exhaling on the downward movement.

Pointers
Again, do not point your toes. Be sure to inhale deeply when performing this exercise.

> *"The bearing and the training of a child is a woman's wisdom."*
>
> —Lord Tennyson

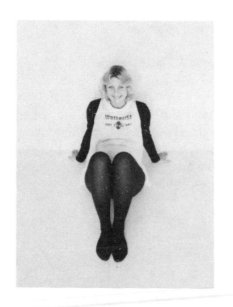

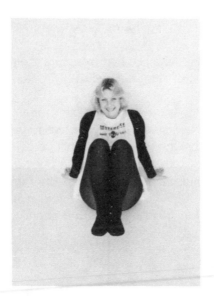

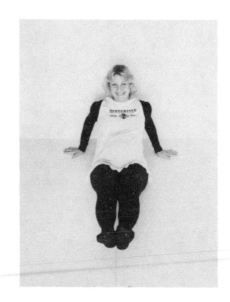

In sitting position, lean back, supporting upper body with arms, and bending knees.

Raise knees towards chest.

Lower and stretch legs.

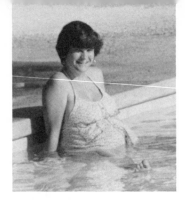

15   The Leg Scissors

Purpose This is the exercise that strengthens your abductor and adductor muscles. The former help your legs to move apart; the latter move your legs together.

Preparation In the supported sitting position (see Strampeln on page 50), with water at bust level, raise your legs until they're level with the floor. Flex your feet to avoid cramps.

Practice Stretch your legs wide apart, keeping them level with the floor and in the water throughout the exercise. Move your legs towards each other, continuing the motion until they cross, right over left. Stretch your legs apart, and once again close them, this time moving your left leg over your right. You have now performed one complete movement. Continue in accordance with the Progress Table.

Pointers Try to stretch your legs a little farther apart with each repetition.

The Complete Prenatal Water Workout Book

"Children are our most valuable natural resource."

—Herbert Hoover

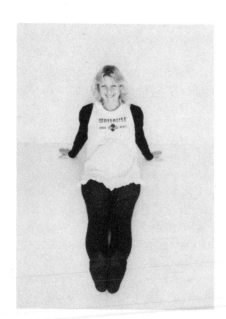

In sitting position, lean back, supporting upper body with arms.

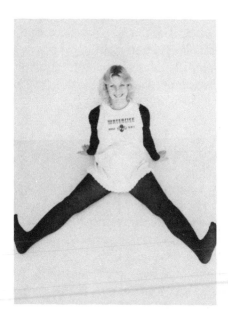

Stretch legs wide apart.

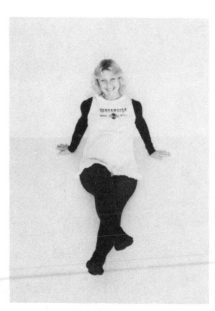

Cross legs in scissor motion.

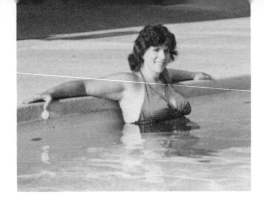

16   The Water Kegel

Purpose   Named after Dr. Arnold Kegel, this most important of all prenatal exercises firms the pelvic floor muscles. The pelvic floor muscles come under considerable stress during pregnancy, particularly when standing. Firming them provides better support for the reproductive organs and helps prevent urinary incontinence (the uncontrolled leaking of urine). This exercise will also restore the stretched vaginal canal to normal size and tone after birth.

Preparation   Stand in chest-high water. Lean backwards against the side of the pool, resting your shoulders against the wall for support. Cross your legs at the ankles.

Practice   After tightening your thigh and buttock muscles, tighten the pelvic floor muscles with the same action you would use to check the flow of urine. Of the three sphincter muscles, the one you will most readily feel is the anal sphincter. Continue tightening so that it feels as if this muscle is being pulled up into the rectum. Hold all of these muscles contracted for the count of two; then relax them *slowly*. Inhale with each contraction and exhale with each relaxation, holding your breath during the count of two. Repeat in accordance with the recommendations in the Progress Table.

Pointers   This exercise may be practiced anywhere, in or out of the water, and is worth continuing as a regular exercise throughout life.

"Motherhood is the greatest role a woman can have."

—Rose Kennedy

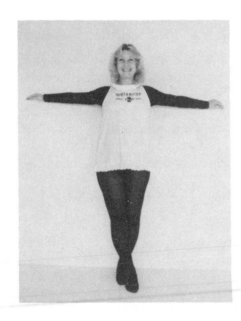

Lean against pool wall with legs crossed.

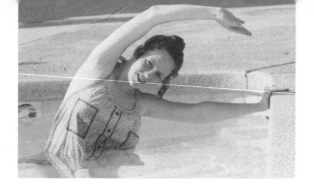

17   Side Bend Side

Purpose   In addition to firming your waist, this exercise helps strengthen your lower back muscles, thereby reducing the backaches that often occur during pregnancy.

Preparation   In waist-high water, stand so that your left side is next to the edge of the pool. Fully extend your left arm, grasping the wall or rail for support. Keep your feet together.

Practice   Curve your right arm over your head, stretching towards the rail and causing your left shoulder to drop. Move your right arm back over your head, fully extending it to the right. Repeat in accordance with the Progress Table. Now repeat the exercise sequence while holding onto the pool with your right hand.

Pointers   Make sure to keep the supporting arm straight, even when the shoulder drops.

The Complete Prenatal Water Workout Book

"The three most beautiful sights . . . a potato garden in bloom, a ship in sail, and a woman after the birth of her child."

—Irish Proverb

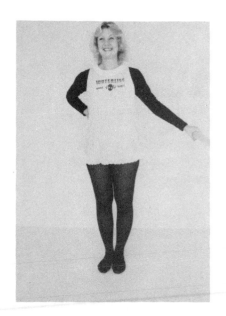

Grasp rail for support.

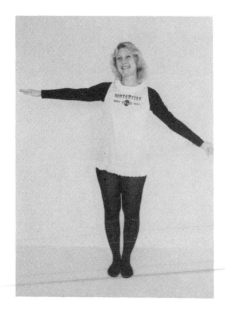

Extend right arm.

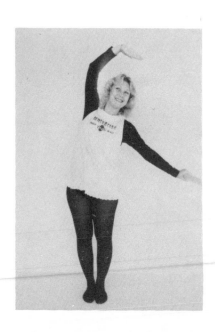

Curve right arm over head, dropping left shoulder.

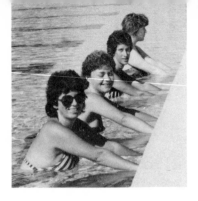

18   Pelvic Water Rock

Purpose   In addition to strengthening the muscles of the abdomen and the lower back, this exercise also loosens the pelvic joints and the lower spine to help prevent backache during pregnancy.

Preparation   In waist-high water, stand about two feet away from the pool's edge, facing the pool wall. Keep your legs comfortably apart. Lean forward slightly, bending at the hip and keeping your back straight. Place your hands on the wall for support.

Practice   Allow your tummy to sag. Lift your tailbone as high as possible while keeping your heels on the floor. Pause; then pull your tailbone down, slightly bend your knees, and tilt your pelvis forward. Do the number of repetitions recommended in the Progress Table.

Pointers   Anticipate a little pain behind your knees as you lift your tailbone.

> *"Mighty is the force of Motherhood! It transforms all things by its vital heart."*
>
> —George Eliot

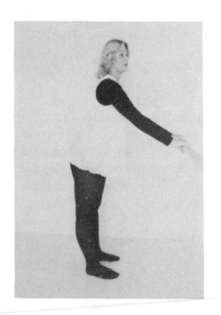 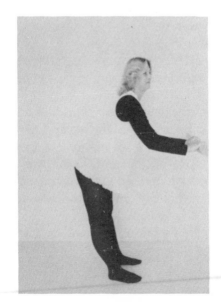 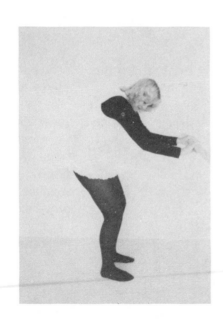

Bend forward at hip, keeping back straight.

Lift tailbone up, allowing tummy to sag.

Pull tailbone down, tilting pelvis forward.

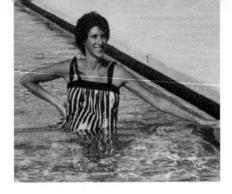

19   Leg Exercises

Purpose   These exercises will strengthen your hip and leg muscles, all of which aid the maintenance of good posture.

Preparation   In waist-high water, stand so that your left side faces the edge of the pool. Grasp the rail or wall with your left hand; place your other hand on your hip.

Practice   Raise your right leg sideways until your toes are as high as is comfortable. If possible, your toes should be just out of the water. Then bring your leg across in front of your body, again raising your toes just out of the water. Return your leg to the side, moving it in a circle on the way. Finish with toes again out of the water. Do the number of repetitions prescribed in the Progress Table. Now repeat the exercise sequence, this time holding onto the pool with your right hand and raising your left leg.

Pointers   Make sure that the thumb of the hand on the hip is pointing forward.

"The yoking of all the powers of the body, mind and soul are needed to prepare for joyful Motherhood."

—Indian Proverb

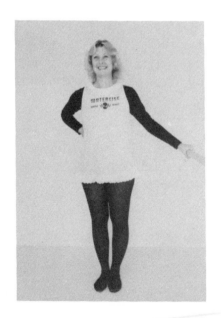

Grasp rail with left hand, and place right hand on hip.

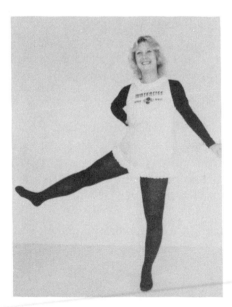

Raise right leg sideways, as high as comfort permits.

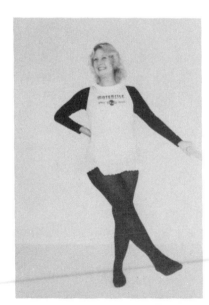

Swing leg across front of body.

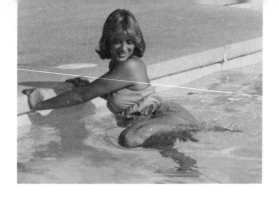

20   The Cellulite Slayer

Purpose   Cellulite tends to cling to the hips and buttocks when surplus fat accumulates on the body. Firming your hip and buttock muscles will help to remove cellulite deposits.

Preparation   With water at chest level, stand facing the side of the pool. Grasp the rail or wall, keeping your arms and body straight. Tilt your body slightly forward towards the side of the pool.

Practice   Raise your right leg straight out behind. Look back over your right shoulder while bending your right knee so that your lower leg moves behind your body, calf parallel to the floor of the pool. Straighten your right leg and resume the starting position. Repeat the sequence with the left leg. Counting the entire sequence as a repetition, do the number recommended in the Progress Table.

Pointers   You may experience a leg cramp if you lift your leg too high on the first movement. If you do, begin again, lifting your leg to a more comfortable height.

"Men are what their mothers made them."

—Ralph Waldo Emerson

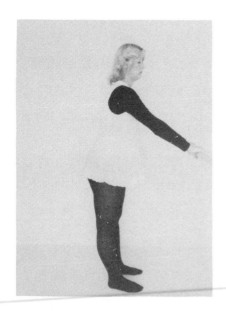 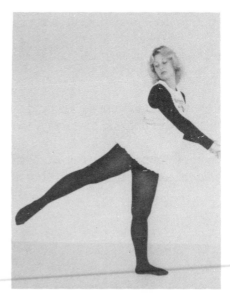 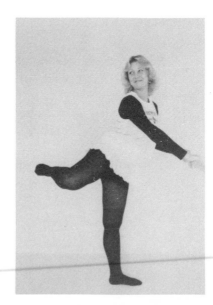

Grasp rail, keeping arms and body straight.

Raise right leg, turning hips.

Bend knee so that calf moves behind body, parallel to floor.

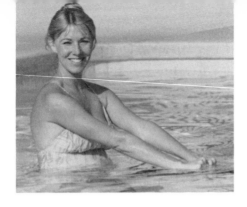

21   Pushing the Stroller

Purpose This general body toning exercise includes isometrics to firm your bust. This exercise will also help you to bond with your unborn child.

Preparation Stand erect in chest-high water, with your arms held out in front, straight and stiff, as if pushing a stroller.

Practice Walk back and forth across the pool, keeping your arms straight. On alternate steps, push your fists together, relaxing them with the next step.

Pointers To receive maximum benefit from the isometric aspect of this exercise, be sure to hold your shoulders well back as you push your fists together.

"My opportunity is here. I will do what I can for all my children."

—Old Aztec Prayer

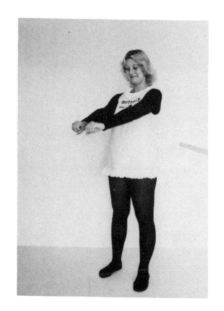

Hold arms straight and stiff.

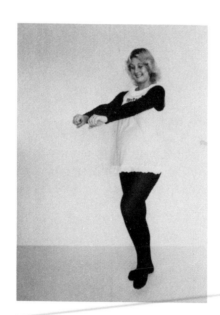

Push that stroller!

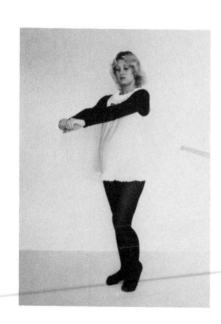

On alternate steps, push fists together.

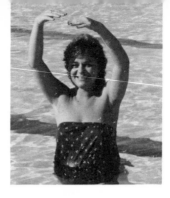

22 Full Deep Breathing

Purpose   Oxygen is absorbed by the muscles during activity. Deep breathing will replace the additional oxygen used while exercising.

Preparation Muscular activity absorbs oxygen. Deep breathing will provide you with the additional oxygen needed while exercising.

Practice   Inhale slowly while raising your arms above your head in an easy sweeping motion, allowing your lungs to fill right up to the top of your chest. Exhale while leaning slightly forward and lowering your arms to a relaxed position. Repeat, this time holding your breath for a count of four when your arms are above your head. Exhale in the manner already described. This complete sequence should be repeated three times.

Pointers   Breathe in through your nose, and out through your mouth.

> *"It's time that people realize that women in this country can do any job that they want to do."*
>
> —Sally Ride

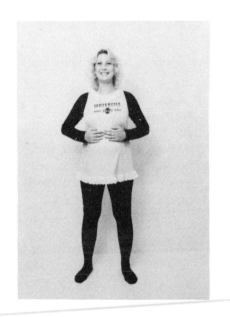

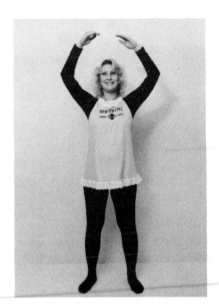

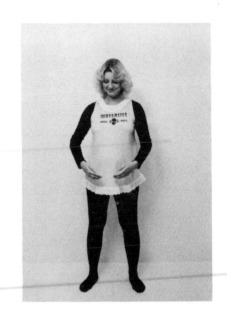

Hold hands against lower ribs.

Raise arms above head.

Lower arms to relaxed position.

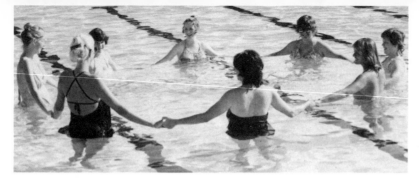

23   Happy Thoughts

Purpose   When *Watercising* with friends, this cooling down exercise creates a bond of togetherness.

Preparation   Stand in waist-high water with legs comfortably apart, forming a circle with your friends.

Practice   Bend your knees until the water is at shoulder level. Lean slightly forward from the waist with your arms outstretched in front, and move your arms in a rowing motion while singing the first line of the rhyme. Next, flutter your fingers through the water while singing the second line. With the third line, straighten up and hold hands with your neighbors, taking two steps to the right and two steps to the left. Release hands for the fourth line, reaching up to the sky with a final stretch while looking up.

The Rhyme: "Row, row, row your boat,
Gently down life's stream.
Merrily, merrily, merrily, merrily,
Stretch, and reach your dream!"

Chapter Six
Shower and Tub Exercises

Whether showering prior to entering a public pool or taking a shower or bath at home, the opportunity to benefit from further simple exercises should not be missed, particulary in view of the water environment.

When practiced in the shower prior to your *Watercise* workout, these exercises will help to release tension and prepare your body for the *Watercise* sequence. The tub exercises will provide a little extra stretching and toning of important muscles. The bathtub is also a good place to practice Retreat Time—especially if your *Watercise* pool is noisy.

In a shower or tub, the use of a massage spray is particularly beneficial, as is the use of a loofah sponge to vitalize the skin. You may find that the prenatal use of Vitamin-E-enriched soaps and body lotions will help reduce stretch marks.

Beware of a slippery floor in the shower, and stand on a rubber shower mat whenever possible. For the tub exercises, an air pillow or small swim float placed behind the back may enhance comfort.

The Neck Soother

Purpose	Tension often causes the neck muscles to partially contract, leading to pain in the neck, head, and back. This exercise is designed to reduce such tension.
Preparation	Stand erect in the shower, with your back to the shower head, feet comfortably apart, and arms hanging limply at your sides.
Practice	Tilt your head gently to the left; then stretch it further by extending your neck slantwise towards the ceiling. Straighten your neck and bend your head forward slightly; then tilt it gently to the left again, stretch, and straighten. Now bend your head back slightly and again tilt to the left, stretch, and straighten. Repeat this three-stage exercise, this time tilting the head to the right. Then complete the entire sequence two more times.
Pointers	The greatest benefit will be obtained if you are able to relax your muscles as you gently stretch your neck.

The Complete Prenatal Water Workout Book

Neck Rotations

Purpose   Neck rotations further stretch the neck muscles to prevent the return of tension.

Preparation   Stand as for the Neck Soother.

Practice   Turn your head gently but fully to the left; then turn it a little farther; then again a bit farther. Return to the starting position, pause, and repeat to the right. Do this exercise three times in each direction.

Pointers   Prevent your shoulders from twisting or dropping during this exercise, as this will decrease the effectiveness of the movement.

Shoulder Circles

Purpose   Although this exercise works the shoulder muscles, its main purpose is to stretch the neck muscles to keep tension at bay. The neck muscles originate in the collarbone and the shoulder blades and insert in the skull. Thus, the downward movement of the shoulder stretches the neck muscles in another direction, helping them to relax.

Preparation   Stand as for the Neck Soother.

Practice   Slowly lift both shoulders—first forwards and upwards, and then backwards. Lift them as high as possible. Continue the slow backwards movement as you start to bring your shoulders downwards, and finally forwards, completing the circle. Complete three circles before reversing direction for three more circles.

Pointers   To obtain maximum benefit from this exercise, avoid moving your trunk from the waist while doing Shoulder Circles.

The Isometric Bust Lifter

Purpose   This exercise strengthens the pectoral muscles, helping to hold a firm bustline.

Preparation   With the tub filled to the regular level, sit upright, with legs and arms stretched straight out in front. Turn palms outward and press lightly against the inside of the tub walls.

Practice   Inhale slowly and deeply, at the same time pushing your hands outwards against the tub. Push and relax your hands four times before exhaling and totally relaxing. Repeat three times.

Pointers   Avoid pushing the length of your arms against the sides of the tub. The effort should be made with your hands only. Keep your toes flexed to avoid cramps.

Preparing for Labor

Purpose The position described in this exercise is considered by many childbirth experts to be the most comfortable and advantageous birth position. Be aware, though, that some doctors and hospitals do not allow women to use the position. Discuss the use of this technique with your doctor. Practice during the *last two months of pregnancy* should lead to a feeling of ease during delivery as well as help to stretch the perineum.

Preparation With tub water at normal level, sit upright, resting against the back of the tub. For added comfort, place an air pillow behind your back.

Practice Keeping your feet on the floor of the tub, draw your knees up and apart. Grasp the underside of each knee with a hand, and as you pull your legs as far apart as they will go, bend your head forward. Repeat twice.

Pointers When your knees are drawn up *and* pulled apart, the soles of your feet will be slightly turned in towards each other, but not, of course, touching.

Chapter Seven
Making Waves Together

THE FATHER'S ROLE DURING PREGNANCY

Throughout this book, I have stressed the importance of successful intrauterine bonding, and have quoted experts who believe that the feelings and experiences of the mother-to-be can be transmitted to her unborn child. Everything a mother does to improve her own mental and physical health also improves the mental and physical health of her unborn child. However, while the expectant mother may be giving her all, the expectant father may be giving little or nothing—even if unintentionally.

What the expectant father does, or does not do, in support of the efforts of his partner can affect his child. Any negative feelings—fear, pain, anger, or resentment—that the father causes in the expectant mother may be felt by the child. But so too can feelings of love, affection, and admiration flow from the father to the mother and on to the child. *An expectant father can imprint on the mind of his unborn child his own feelings of love and adoration.*

Many believe that the unborn child can sense outside noises during the last three or four months of pregnancy, and that the child may be able to recognize these sounds after birth. The father who lovingly talks to his unborn child may be rewarded by his child's early recognition of him after birth.

Undoubtedly, gentle fun and games between partners will transmit positive feelings to the child, as will togetherness in any joyous form. I suggest that you ask your partner to read this book before he joins you in the togetherness exercises that follow.

When doing these informal exercises together, splash a little, laugh a little, and enjoy yourselves.

Storking Together

To stork together, stand side by side with arms placed around your partner's waist, as you may have done for a three-legged race at school. Each of you should then raise your *outer* leg to begin *storking* in the manner described in the Stork Walk on page 30. Continue for as long as you wish.

Holding Hands Together

Stand facing each other in waist-high water. To avoid bumping during exercising, each of you should take a half step sideways to the right. Reach out, gripping each other's hands, left hand to partner's right, right hand to partner's left. Now begin the sequence, holding hands throughout all five exercises.

1. With feet comfortably apart and turned out, do ten half squats, forcing the knees wide apart as you lower your body, and pulling them together as you rise.

2. Stand erect with feet a few inches apart. With foot flexed, raise your right leg forward and upward. Then swing your leg back down and out to the right in a continuous motion before bringing it down again. Repeat ten times before moving a full step to the left and repeating the exercise with your left leg.

3. Stand erect with feet a few inches apart. Lift your left leg forward to a comfortable height and, without pointing your toes, rotate your foot in a small circle five times. Now swing your left leg to the rear, again

to a comfortable height, and make five circles. Take a full step to the right and repeat the exercise with your right leg.

4. Stand erect with feet a few inches apart. Lift your right foot and slide it up your left leg to the top of the calf, allowing the knee to swing out sideways. Now kick to the right before bringing your foot back to standing position. Repeat ten times. Then take a full step to the left and repeat with your left leg.

5. Stand erect with feet a few inches apart. Take a half step to the right so that you again face each other. Raise your left leg backwards, bending it at the knee to bring your heel as close to your buttocks as possible. Repeat ten times with each leg.

Retreating Together

When parents-to-be share intimate moments, there exists a special feeling of togetherness and tenderness. When those moments are spent in peaceful relaxation, meditation, and visualization of their forming child, the feeling of togetherness has no bounds.

After exercising together, take a few moments more to retreat together from the outside world and to focus on the precious life within the womb. The aim is much the same as for Retreat Time, but the technique is different. And, of course, you will be sharing this time with your partner.

Move together into chest-high water, where the expectant father can support you while you float on your back. His left hand should be under the small of your back, and his right hand on top of your stomach. Close your eyes. The father should look first at your face as you relax, and then at your stomach as he visualizes the child within. Continue to relax, feeling the water gently lap around you as you inhale and exhale to the rhythm of the water. Feel the energy flow from your partner's hands into your body and to your unborn child—a child who is floating as weightlessly and effortlessly in the womb as you are floating in the water. With each exhalation, shed more of your fears and worries, mentally seeing them flow out of your mind and sink to the bottom of the water.

Together, focus on the developing mind of your child, and resolve to give that child all of the blessings of life. Resolve to teach your child true ideals. Allow your minds to float as if all is within your power and there can be no limitations on your achievements. Visualize how your efforts and abilities will provide your child with the gifts of love, compassion, tolerance, strength, knowledge, and application. See your child become what you both *want* your child to become.

The father should gently break the reverie by slowly caressing your stomach. Open your eyes to find him looking into them as he lifts you gently to your feet.

Leave the pool together, arm in arm, feeling the strength of the bond between you, and knowing that the most beautiful and satisfying time of your lives lies ahead.

Give it all you have, and the rewards will be great. I promise.

Recommended Reading

Brazelton, T. Berry, MD. *Infants and Mothers*. New York: Delta Books/Seymour Lawrence, 1983.

Brinkley, Ginny; Goldberg, Linda; and Kukar, Janice. *Your Child's First Journey: A Guide to Prepared Birth From Pregnancy to Parenthood*. 2nd ed. Garden City Park, NY: Avery Publishing Group, Inc., 1988.

Brown, Nancie Mae. "Rock-a-Bye Your Baby." In *The Holistic Health Handbook*. Berkeley: And/Or Press, Inc., 1978.

Cronin, Isaac, and Brewer, Sforza Gail. *Eating for Two*. New York: Bantam Books, Inc., 1983.

Curtis, Lindsay R., MD. *Pregnant and Loving It*. Tucson: HP Books, 1977.

Dick-Read, Grantly, MD. *Childbirth Without Fear*. 2nd ed. New York: Harper and Row Publishers, Inc., 1953.

Gold, Cybele, and Gold, E.J. "Natural Childbirth." In *The Holistic Health Handbook*. Berkeley: And/Or Press, Inc., 1978.

La Leche League International. *The Womanly Art of Breastfeeding*. New York: New American Library, 1984.

McGarey, Gladys T., MD. *Born to Live*. Phoenix: Gabriel Press, 1980.

Montagu, Ashley. *Life Before Birth*. New York: New American Library, 1965.

Olkin, Sylvia Klein. *Positive Pregnancy Fitness: A Guide to a More Comfortable Pregnancy and Easier Birth Through Exercise and Relaxation.* Garden City Park, NY: Avery Publishing Group, Inc., 1987.

Thevenin, Tine. *The Family Bed: An Age-Old Concept in Child Rearing.* Garden City Park, NY: Avery Publishing Group, 1987.

Verny, Thomas, MD. *The Secret Life of the Unborn Child.* New York: Dell Publishing Co., Inc., 1986.

Woessner, Candace; Lauwers, Judith; and Bernard, Barbara. *Breastfeeding Today: A Mother's Companion.* Garden City Park, NY: Avery Publishing Group, Inc., 1987.

About the Author

Helga Hughes received her early physical exercise training, as well as nutrition and culinary training, at a private girl's college in Forchheim, Bavaria.

Later, in the United States, she became a consultant at the House of Venus Health Spa, and manager of the Elaine Powers Figure Salon, both in Fort Wayne, Indiana.

Following a break during 1972 when she became the first female pilot to graduate from the School of Executive Aviation at Baerfield, Indiana, and then worked as an active "Ninety Niner" in the Womans Pilots International Organization, she moved to the Sun Belt.

In Phoenix, she spent five years as the Recreation and Social Director at Ahwatukee, a major retirement center, where she devised and taught a specialized program called "Slim and Trim Water Exercises." This program was later extended to Leisure World, another major retirement community with locations in Arizona and California.

Benefiting from extensive world travel, Helga is a free-lance writer who covers international cuisine, nutrition, and infant-related subjects, as well as water exercises.

Currently residing in Sandbridge, Virginia, she is working on a new postnatal exercise program.

Helga is a member of the International Childbirth Education Association, the Minneapolis-based organization that supports family-centered maternity care.

Index

Childbirth Books From **Avery**

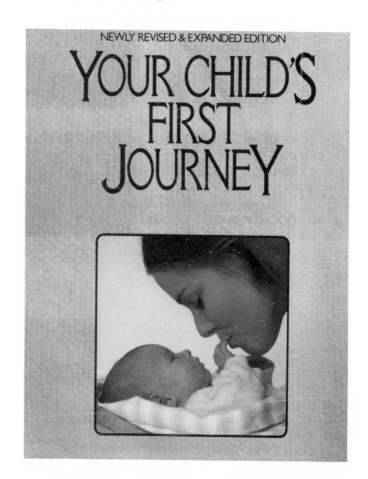

Your Child's First Journey, Second Edition
A Guide to Prepared Birth from Pregnancy to Parenthood
Ginny Brinkley, Linda Goldberg and Janice Kukar

Here is the revised and expanded edition of one of the most widely
used and medically accepted pregnancy guides in the U.S. This
complete, fully illustrated book is written with an emphasis on the
emotional and physical benefits of family-centered care, and on the
importance of being an educated consumer.
This comprehensive text encompasses all of the topics discussed in
Early Pregnancy, Lamaze, Cesarean Preparation, and New Mothers'
classes. Each section contains detailed coverage of an important
aspect of pregnancy, birth, or infant care. Readers gain an
awareness of current trends and controversies as they learn to make
use of the most up-to-date childbirth techniques, and to become
confident and capable parents.
Your Child's First Journey contains a wealth of checklists, step-by-
step guides, and other special features that summarize and
highlight important information. The book is enhanced with well
over 100 photos and illustrations, and is enlivened with cartoons
that provide humorous insights into the feelings and experiences of
the new parent.

$10.95
272 pages
8½ x 11 inch format
Quality paperback
0-89529-372-2

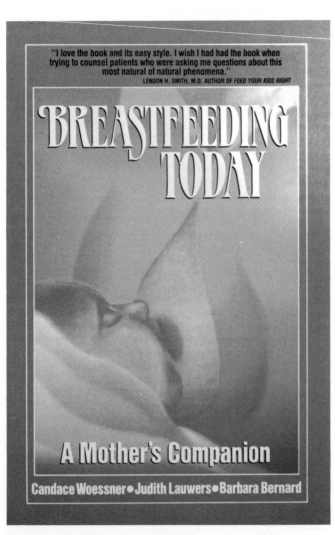

"I love the book and its easy style. I wish I had had the book when trying to counsel patients who were asking me questions about this most natural of natural phenomena."

LENDON H. SMITH, M.D. AUTHOR OF *FEED YOUR KIDS RIGHT*

BREASTFEEDING TODAY

A Mother's Companion

Candace Woessner • Judith Lauwers • Barbara Bernard

Breastfeeding Today

The Mother's Companion

Candace Woessner, Judith Lauwers and Barbara Bernard

Breastfeeding Today is *the* authoritative guide to breastfeeding for today's parents. Written by the authors of the most widely used professional breastfeeding handbook in the country, *Breastfeeding Today* accurately reflects the needs and expectations of today's nursing mother.

Breastfeeding Today explains all aspects of nursing in a style that is warm, reassuring, and easy to read. Parents are guided through the many challenges of today's busy world. From the use of microwave ovens to thaw bottled breast milk to the management of time for the working mother, *Breastfeeding Today* provides the right blend of practical advice and up-to-date information.

Standing apart from all other breastfeeding books, *Breastfeeding Today* is in tune with the way women really live their lives.

$8.95
256 pages
6 x 9 inch format
Quality paperback
0-89529-351-X

Positive Pregnancy Fitness
A Guide to a More Comfortable Pregnancy and Easier Birth
Sylvia Klein Olkin, M.S.

Proper nutrition, daily exercise, and relaxation all add up to a healthy mother — and a healthy baby! Keeping in good physical shape is always important, but particularly so during the pregnant months. *Positive Pregnancy Fitness* by Sylvia Klein Olkin will shape up and energize the pregnant woman and — what's more — show her how to get back into shape after the birth.
Written by the director of the Positive Pregnancy and Parenting Fitness program, who is also an experienced self-development teacher and childbirth educator, *Positive Pregnancy Fitness* presents a safe, effective, and easy-to-learn wholistic program that is already being used successfully by over 10,000 women.
The book contains safe, daily exercise routines based on stress management, body awareness, visualization, and other disciplines that will increase pregnancy comfort and prepare the body for labor. In addition, clear and instructive illustrations enable the reader to see and imitate the various positions.

$9.95
226 pages
8 x 10 inch format
Quality paperback
0-89529-373-0

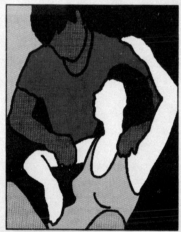

A Guide to a More Comfortable Pregnancy and Easier Birth Through Exercise and Relaxation

POSITIVE
Pregnancy
FITNESS

Sylvia Klein Olkin

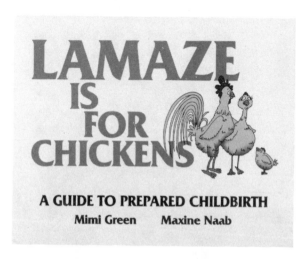

Lamaze Is for Chickens
A Guide to Prepared Childbirth
Mimi Green and Maxine Naab

Designed as a complete guide to Lamaze childbirth, this book — which focuses on the birth process — emphasizes the satisfaction and exhilaration that results from the use of prepared childbirth methods. The authors maintain that childbirth, much like swimming, is a learned skill, requiring training and practice in order for it to be approached with eagerness and joy, rather than fear and trepidation.

Lamaze Is for Chickens provides readers with the necessary training, and guides them through the necessary practice.

$8.95
200 pages
10 x 7¾ inch format
Quality paperback
0-89529-181-9

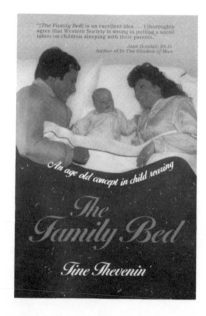

The Family Bed
An Age-Old Concept in Child Rearing
Tine Thevenin

The sharing of the family bed by parents and their children is no modern notion. From cave to castle, all over the world, group sleeping was accepted as the norm. It has only been within the last 150 years that modern Western "authorities" have discouraged this practice. Now there is a book that puts this age-old concept into perspective. *The Family Bed* explores the pros and cons, the joys and irritations that occur when children sleep with their parents. What emerges from this book is a way to solve nighttime problems with young children and a means of creating a closer bond between family members, giving children a greater sense of security.

The Family Bed is a new look at an old idea whose time has come — again.

$7.95
176 pages
6 x 9 inch format
Quality paperback
0-89529-357-9

Our Family Grows

A Coloring & Activity Book
Renee Neri

Beautifully designed to prepare and involve the young child whose mother will soon be giving birth. Includes cut-outs, pictures for coloring, and creative activities for the sister- or brother-to-be. Large type, simple instructions, and amusing cartoons allow the child to have hours and hours of constructive fun. The time spent coloring, cutting, and drawing in *Our Family Grows* will enable the child to share the excitement and joy of having a baby.

$3.95
48 pages
8½ x 11 inch format
Quality paperback
0-89529-299-8

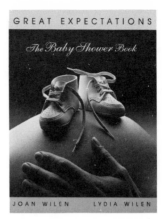

Great Expectations— A Baby Shower Book

Joan Wilen
Lydia Wilen

Here is a unique and novel way of recording the memories of your baby shower. *Great Expectations: A Baby Shower Book* invites family and friends to write down their predictions about the baby, give advice to the mother-to-be, and share their good wishes. Once the pages are filled, the book can be read to all, creating a fun and loving atmosphere.

Just as every mother-to-be has great expectations, so should every baby shower have *Great Expectations*.

$6.95
82 pages
8½ x 11 inch format
Quality paperback
0-89529-247-5

Avery Publishing Group

89 Baldwin Terrace
Wayne, New Jersey 07470

Please make your check or money order payable to Avery Publishing Group, Inc. NY and NJ residents add appropriate sales tax.

Your group or organization may qualify for group quantity discounts. Please write for further information to Customer Service Department, Avery Pubishing Group, 89 Baldwin Terrace, Wayne, NJ 07470.

ORDER FORM

Name_____

Address_____

City _____ State _____ Zip _____

Qty.	Title	Cost Per Book	Amount
		Handling	$1.50
		Total	

7/01 SC NOLAD